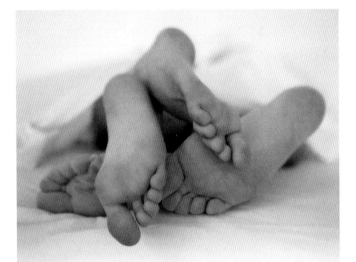

fertility &
conception

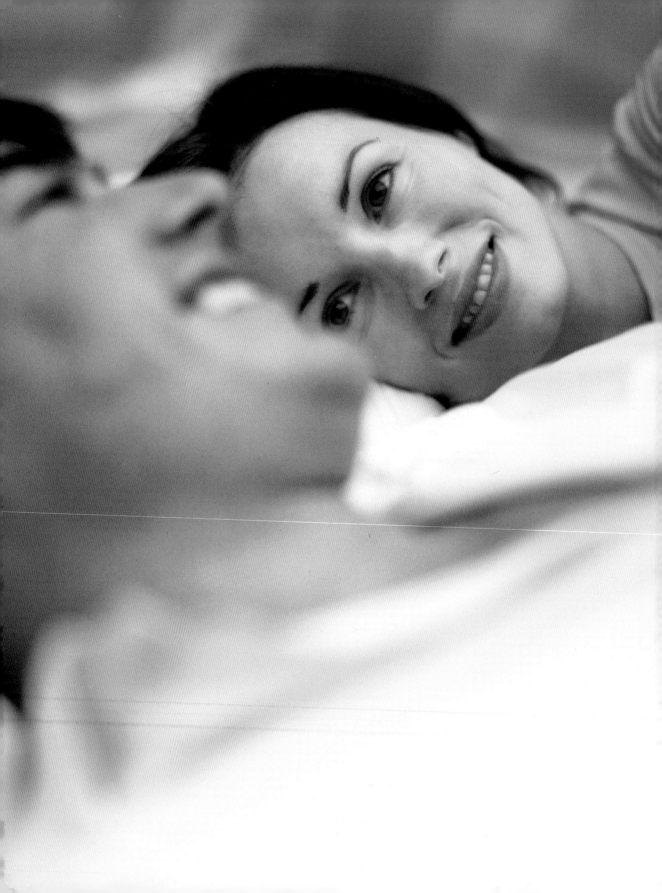

fertility &
conception
the complete guide to getting pregnant

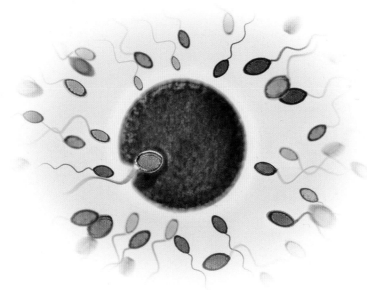

ZITA WEST

DK

LONDON, NEW YORK, MUNICH, MELBOURNE, DELHI

Zita West would like to dedicate this book to
all the clients she has helped over the years

DK LONDON
Senior editor Salima Hirani
Project editor Jude Garlick
Art editor Nicola Rodway
Designer Ann Burnham
DTP designer Karen Constanti
Production controller Mandy Inness
Managing editor Anna Davidson
Managing art editor Emma Forge
Picture researcher Franziska Marking
Jacket designer Chris Drew
Art director Carole Ash
Publisher Corinne Roberts

UPDATED EDITION
Editor Julia Halford
Project editor Martha Burley
Senior art editor Sara Robin
Pre-producer Raymond Williams
Managing editor Dawn Henderson
Creative publishing manager Anna Davidson
Managing art editor Christine Keilty
Art director Jane Bull
Publisher Peggy Vance

DK INDIA
Senior editor Nidhilekha Mathur
Senior designer Ira Sharma
Senior DTP designers Pushpak Tyagi, Tarun Sharma
Managing editor Alicia Ingty
Managing art editor Navidita Thapa
Pre-production manager Sunil Sharma

First published in Great Britain in 2003 by Dorling Kindersley Limited,
80 Strand, London WC2R 0RL

Penguin Group (UK)

This updated edition published in Great Britain in 2014

Copyright © 2003, 2014 Dorling Kindersley Limited

Text copyright © 2003, 2014 Zita West

2 4 6 8 10 9 7 5 3 1

ISBN: 978 1 4093 4677 7

Reproduced by Colourscan, Singapore

Printed and bound by Leo Paper Product Ltd., China

Discover more at **www.dk.com**

Contents

Chapter 4
Testing your fertility

Chapter 5
Assisted conception

**Sperm in a
Fallopian tube.**

Author's introduction

Do you see yourself with a baby? This is a question I ask all my clients when they come to the clinic.

A vast majority of couples can have a baby. It depends on how far they are prepared to go to achieve it. Every couple is different in terms of what they are willing to consider, from natural conception to IVF, egg donation, surrogacy and adoption.

My vocation is as a midwife; my deep commitment to fertility has come from that role. My passion is helping couples to focus on, plan for and succeed in having a baby. It is a wonderful privilege to work with a couple prior to conception, get a positive pregnancy result, and look after them during pregnancy and birth.

My approach has its roots in long-held Chinese beliefs. These are based on knowledge of the human body that came from listening and observing and understanding natural laws and fertility cycles. They incorporate key principles of fertility that we have moved away from today. In this book you will find many simple measures combined with the very latest Western technology, making the most of ancient and modern.

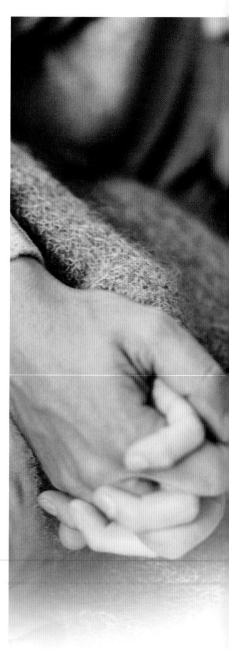

Helping couples to conceive requires a focused, planned, common-sense approach. My pregnancy plan starts with an organized attempt at natural conception. I often find that couples are willing to make radical changes to their lives and consider expending a great deal of time, energy, money and emotion on elaborate treatments, but they may, for example, simply be having sex at the wrong time or be unaware of the intricacies of the female reproductive cycle.

I believe that fertility awareness, nutrition and lifestyle are key. We'll look at your nutrition, but faddy diets and mega-doses of supplements are not necessary. Follow an eating plan that suits you, but in moderation. I see couples who

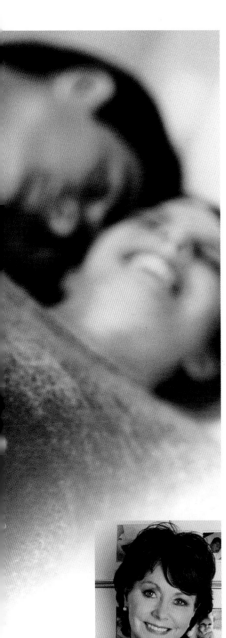

have all but given up their normal habits, and feel as if life is almost not worth living. Don't beat yourself up about the odd glass of wine or cup of coffee you have had this month – the stress won't help you conceive. I provide many tips on how to adjust your lifestyle, but again, becoming obsessive is not an effective way of achieving conception.

If you have given all the natural methods your best shot, and you're still not pregnant, you can move on to a plan for assisted conception. I'll take you through all the options, with in-depth coverage of one of the most common fertility treatments – in vitro fertilization, or IVF. Preparing for IVF is the same as preparing for any pregnancy, and you should regard your treatment as part of a process, not a one-off event.

I am strongly in favour of appropriate complementary techniques to enhance fertility and conception, but I believe in an evidence-based approach. Couples need support and positive expectation, not false hope. Complementary medicine should work in conjunction with Western medicine. There are many good therapists and treatments out there, but beware of ignorance among practitioners about fertility and the "psychobabble" of some therapists.

There are many factors affecting conception today that we have only recently come to appreciate, and modern trends in fertility give couples a lot to think about. Whatever you are faced with, remember, focus; don't give up everything; don't put your life on hold.

I do hope this book helps you to get closer to your goal of having a baby.

Zita West

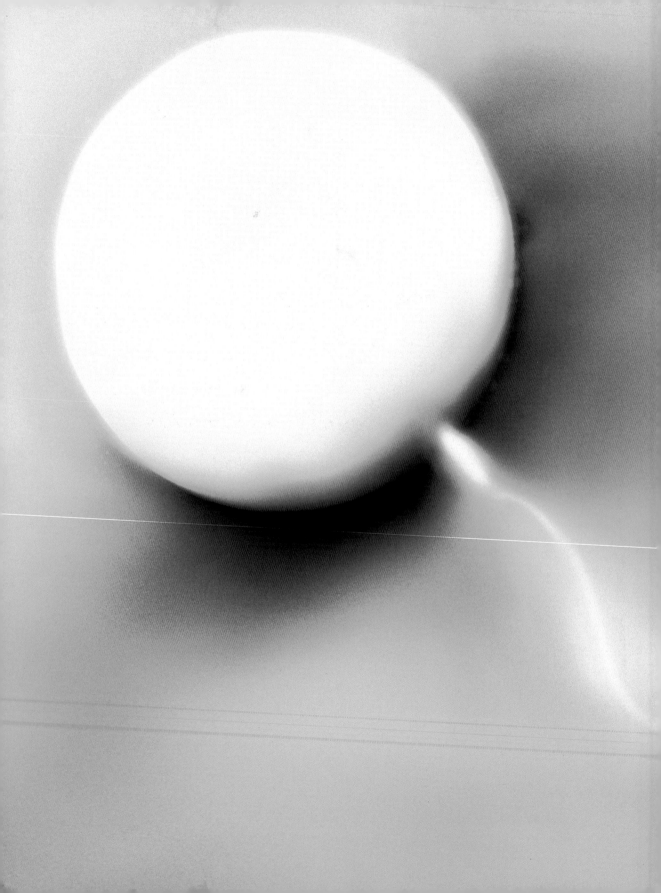

Fertility facts

Many women and men don't think much about reproduction and fertility until they want a baby. *You would be surprised* at just how many couples I see do not fully appreciate how their systems work. *In knowledge lies the ability* to improve your own chances of conception. *The starting points* are the basic details of the female and male reproductive systems and how they relate to the all-important issue of fertility and ageing.

Reproduction in women

A woman's supply of eggs – several million initially – is created while she herself is in the womb. By puberty, between a quarter and half a million remain. During her life only 400 or so of those will be released via ovulation.

Hormones and the cycle

The ovaries are roughly the size of small plums and they contain a lifetime's supply of immature eggs. Each month, an egg develops to maturity and is released from one ovary, ready for fertilization. The ovaries also produce oestrogen and progesterone.

The average menstrual cycle is 28 days long and has two distinct phases. The first is the follicular phase, associated with the production of oestrogen which stimulates the egg to develop within the ovary until it is released (ovulation). The second is the luteal phase, associated with progesterone. During this phase the womb lining grows so that a fertilized egg can implant in it and be nourished.

The follicular phase

The first day of the menstrual cycle is the first day of bleeding (see page 12), which marks the start of the follicular phase. This is when the egg (ovum) grows and develops. Every female is born with some 2 million eggs, although only 300–400 will mature and be released during her lifetime. The nucleus of the ovum contains half the genetic material (chromosomes) needed to produce a new individual – the other half comes from the sperm.

At the start of the follicular phase, the hypothalamus in the brain (which regulates the pituitary gland) releases gonadotrophin releasing hormone (GnRH). This signals to the pituitary gland to release follicle-stimulating hormone (FSH), which stimulates the eggs inside the ovary to grow. About 20 immature eggs respond and begin to develop within sacs known as follicles, which provide the nourishment the eggs need to grow.

As the eggs develop, the ovaries release oestrogen. This hormone signals to the pituitary gland to reduce FSH production so that only enough is released to stimulate one egg to continue developing. The rest shrivel away. Oestrogen also stimulates the lining of the uterus (endometrium) to begin to thicken, preparing it for implantation of the fertilized egg. The primary follicle contains the egg that has grown most rapidly. Once mature, it is about half the size of a grain of sand and is the largest cell in the human body.

The body's oestrogen level continues to rise until it triggers a surge of luteinizing hormone (LH) from the pituitary gland. This stimulates ovulation, whereby the follicle ruptures and the egg is gently released along with its follicular fluid on to the surface of the ovary.

The luteal phase

Having released the egg, the ruptured follicle continues to receive pulses of LH. This enables it to turn into a small cyst known as the corpus

Crystals of oestradiol, a naturally occuring oestrogen.

A mature human egg just before ovulation.

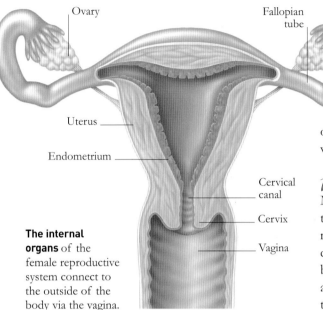

Ovary

Fallopian tube

Uterus

Endometrium

Cervical canal

Cervix

Vagina

The internal organs of the female reproductive system connect to the outside of the body via the vagina.

muscular contractions, help to move the ovum along the tube to the uterus. The journey from the ovary to the uterus takes about six days. The egg will never complete this journey if it is not fertilized: instead it disintegrates and is absorbed. Fertilization needs to occur within 24 hours of ovulation, making the window of opportunity quite short.

Fertilization

Most healthy sperm live in the female reproductive tract for three to five (and up to seven) days, which means that intercourse can take place up to seven days before ovulation and fertilization will still be possible. Cervical secretions act as a barrier to abnormal sperm, which are unable to swim up the channels in the secretions. This ensures that only strong, well-formed sperm make it through the cervix and uterus to the Fallopian tube. The journey from ejaculation to the Fallopian tube takes 30–60 minutes, with many barriers along the way. It is a distance of only 10cm (4in).

An egg is about 550 times wider than the tiny sperm head, so it presents a large target. The sperm's first task when it reaches the egg is to get through the cumulus oophorous. Only good-quality, motile sperm are able do this and many of them die in the process. The sperm then has to attach to the egg and penetrate the zona pellucida. This is a major barrier, four times thicker than the head of the sperm. The release of solubilizing enzymes and a change in the sperm's swimming technique – lashing its tail 800 times a second to generate sufficient force – allow it to penetrate this barrier within about four hours. Most sperm fail to attach and simply bounce off. The zona pellucida thus encourages the strongest and healthiest sperm to penetrate the egg successfully.

luteum, whose job is to produce progesterone. Progesterone has three important functions: it builds and thickens the endometrium, developing glandular structures and blood vessels that supply nutrients to the developing embryo; and it switches off production of FSH and LH. It also raises the basal body temperature (BBT) by about 0.2°C (32.4°F), warming the uterus ready for a fertilized egg.

The journey of the egg

The egg is surrounded by a protective shell known as the zona pellucida. This in turn is surrounded by a mass of sticky cells known as the cumulus oophorous. These cells allow the fimbriae, finger-like projections at the end of each Fallopian tube, to pick up the egg and sweep it into the tube.

A Fallopian tube is roughly the diameter of a pencil, with a narrow channel within it leading from the fimbriae to the uterus. The channel is lined with microscopic hairs called cilia which, together with

The lining of the Fallopian tube.

The lining of the uterus (endometrium) at mid-cycle.

Once the shell is breached, the sperm sheds its tail so that only the head, the part containing the genetic information, fuses with the nucleus of the egg. The fertilized egg now contains a full complement of 46 chromosomes, which it needs to develop into a fully functioning, complete human being. A chemical reaction in the egg immediately hardens the zona pellucida so that no more sperm can get in. Cell division begins.

The fertilized egg, which is known as a zygote at this stage of development, divides into two after 36 hours (on average). It generally has four cells within 46 hours and eight cells within 54–56 hours of fertilization. The rapidly developing embryo travels along the Fallopian tube for the next few days until it reaches the uterus, nourished by mucus secreted by cells in the lining of the tube.

If fertilization does not occur, the egg is absorbed by the body. Without production of the pregnancy hormone human chorionic gonadotrophin (HCG – see below), progesterone levels will fall. The endometrium begins to disintegrate, the uterus sheds the broken blood tissue through the vagina (menstruation) and the cycle begins again.

Implantation

Since ovulation, as a result of a signal from luteinizing hormone (LH), a number of changes have been taking place in the lining of the uterus ready for implantation. Specialized structures called pinopodes develop in cells within the endometrium, creating the ideal conditions for implantation.

They remove fluid from the uterine cavity to ensure good contact between the embryo and the maternal surface. The endometrium also secretes proteins that aid attachment.

By the time it reaches the uterus, the embryo has about 30 cells and is known as a blastocyst. It now starts to break out of the zona pellucida. As women age, the zona becomes tougher, making it more difficult for the embryo to hatch out. IVF (in vitro fertilization) procedures may include assisted hatching, whereby the shell is broken slightly to help the embryo to emerge.

The embryo arrives in the uterus about 4–5 days after fertilization. By this stage the endometrium is about 10mm (½in) thick. The more developed the blastocyst before it implants, the greater the chance of a successful pregnancy.

Implantation is aided by the uterus, which presses its back and front walls together over the embryo rather like a closed fist, holding it firmly in place until it is safely embedded in the endometrium. Part of the growing embryo soon makes contact with the mother's blood supply.

The attachment of the embryo to the endometrium stimulates the production of the pregnancy hormone HCG. This is the hormone that is detected by tests to confirm pregnancy. It stimulates the corpus luteum to continue to produce progesterone to maintain the pregnancy until the placenta produces sufficient progesterone to take over (by the 12th week of pregnancy). This then takes over the role of producing progesterone.

Sperm try to penetrate the thick surface of an egg in order to fuse with the egg nucleus.

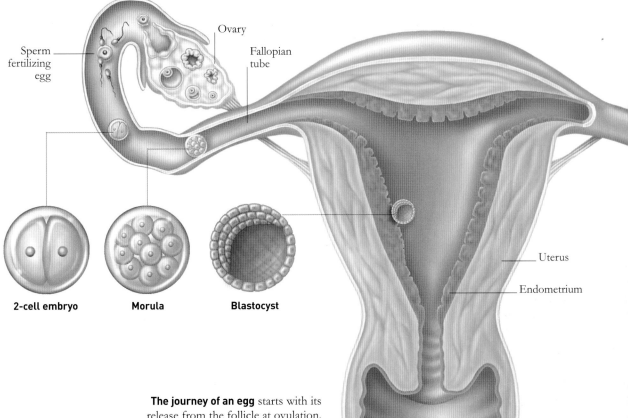

Sperm
fertilizing
egg

Ovary

Fallopian
tube

Uterus

Endometrium

2-cell embryo   **Morula**   **Blastocyst**

The journey of an egg starts with its
release from the follicle at ovulation.
It passes along the Fallopian tube and, if
fertilization occurs, implants in the uterus.

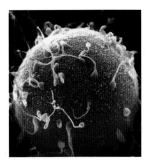

During fertilization,
the sperm – seen here
as hair-like structures –
attempt to penetrate the
thick surface of the egg
in order to fuse with its
nucleus. Only one sperm
will be successful in
doing this.

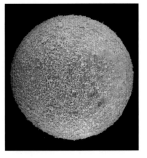

A zygote is a fertilized egg
– this is what it looks like
one day after fertilization.
This primitive embryo
contains all the genetic
material inherited from
the father's sperm and the
mother's ovum. It is about
to start cell division.

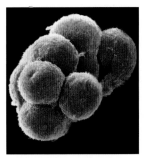

A morula is an embryo
about four days after
fertilization. There has
been a series of cell
divisions by this time and
there are about 12–16 cells
present. The cells are
enclosed by a very thin
protein layer.

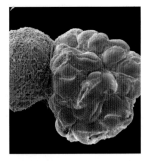

The blastocyst stage occurs
at about five days after
fertilization. The embryo
can be seen "hatching"
from a hole in the zona
pellucida. At this stage
an embryo consists of
at least 30 cells and may
have many more.

Reproduction in men

Men are producing sperm all the time. From puberty, they manufacture sperm constantly – an adult male produces many millions of them every day.

Hormones and sperm production

Hormonal processes are similar in men and women. In both, the hypothalamus releases gonadotrophin-releasing hormone (GnRH). This occurs every 60–90 minutes in men, triggering the pituitary gland to release follicle-stimulating hormone (FSH) and luteinizing hormone (LH). A man produces FSH and LH at an even rate throughout the month, enabling sperm cells to be produced and matured constantly. So in theory, he is always fertile. This fertility does, however, depend upon a perfect balance between FSH and LH being maintained at all times.

Luteinizing hormone stimulates the leydig cells in the testes to produce testosterone. This hormone plays a very important part in several reproductive (among other) functions, including sexual arousal, the production of seminal fluid and the maturation of sperm.

The testes are roughly the same size as the ovaries and are located in the scrotal sac outside the body. They are made up of thousands of tiny coiled tubes known as seminiferous tubules. FSH stimulates spermatocytes – primary sperm cells within the tubules – to divide and develop into spermatids – young, tail-less sperm. The spermatids develop here over a 72-day period, nourished by the sertoli cells lining the tubules.

During this period, each spermatid grows a head containing genetic material (chromosomes), a middle piece containing materials that generate energy for the sperm's movement, and a tail.

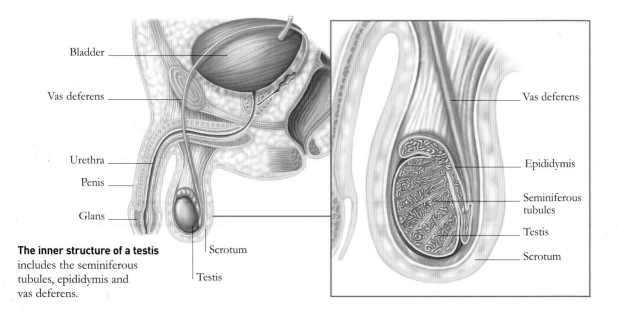

Bladder

Vas deferens

Urethra

Penis

Glans

Scrotum

Testis

The inner structure of a testis includes the seminiferous tubules, epididymis and vas deferens.

Vas deferens

Epididymis

Seminiferous tubules

Testis

Scrotum

Acrosome cap

The sperm's very long tail helps to propel it forwards.

Head   Midpiece   Tail

When the sperm is almost fully mature, it leaves the tubules and enters the epididymis, a long coiled tube attached to the back of a testicle. This tube is an astonishing 6m (20ft) in length, but only one three-hundredth of an inch in diameter.

Sperm and semen

It takes several days for sperm to move along the length of the epididymis and develop full motility, the ability to beat their tails to propel them forward and swim in a straight line rather than round in circles. The sperm then move into the vas deferens to await ejaculation. This tube has a huge capacity – it may take about 30 ejaculations to empty the vas deferens of its full load.

The first contractions of orgasm come from the epididymis and the vas deferens, and these move sperm up into the urethra. En route, the seminal vesicles and other male accessory glands contract violently, expelling fluid. Muscular contractions of the penis then move the ejaculate (semen), which consists of the sperm plus the fluids, forcefully out through the end of the penis.

Sperm form less than 20 per cent of the volume of ejaculate. The composition of semen includes more than 22 different chemicals, including fructose (sugar), vitamins B12, C and E, the minerals potassium, sulphur and zinc, prostaglandins and other (essential) fatty acids.

Ejaculation

Seminal fluid is ejaculated as a viscous, coagulated mass (coagulum) that usually liquefies after about 10 minutes. This protects the sperm in the hostile, acidic environment of the vagina and provides them with energy (after liquefaction) so that they have the power to swim through the cervical mucus to find

Facts about sperm

* 380 cell divisions are needed to make one sperm, compared with only 23 cell divisions required to produce one egg.
* Up to 1,500 sperm per second are produced within each testicle.
* Sperm swim at a rate of 3mm (⅛in) per hour.
* Even if a man ejaculates up to 300 million sperm at a time, only about one million of them make it as far as the cervix. Two hundred at most will reach a Fallopian tube and therefore have a chance of fertilizing an egg.

an egg and then to cling on to it. About 250 million sperm are ejaculated at one time. Why so many? Because they face the prospect of an incredible journey that has very many obstacles along the way. The chances are that relatively few sperm, even out of millions, will have the strength or level of fitness to complete the journey to the egg successfully.

These sperm are passing along a tube in the rete testis. This tube links the seminiferous tubules with the vas deferens.

Age and fertility

Female age is very important in consideration of probability for conception. Male age is less important, although age does have some impact on male fertility.

Things to consider

There are several crucially important factors to consider when you are assessing your fertility and whether or not your age will make a difference.

Ovarian reserve The so-called biological clock has a significant impact on a woman's fertility. A woman is born with all the eggs she will ever have. Her

Statistics

The older the couple, the more difficult it becomes for them to conceive. A study in 2002 explored the average conception figures for healthy women over a one-year period. It found that:

* **by age 24**, 86% of couples were likely to conceive
* **by age 29**, 78% of couples were likely to conceive
* **by age 34**, 63% of couples were likely to conceive
* **by age 39**, 52% of couples were likely to conceive
* **by age 44**, 36% of couples were likely to conceive.

AGEING AND FEMALE FERTILITY

Declining fertility is more of an issue for women than men. Assuming that ovulation occurs normally, that sexual intercourse takes place at the right time and there are no medical or health problems, statistics show that:

* **at the age of 15**, a woman has a 40–50% chance of conceiving per cycle
* **at 25**, she has a 30–35% chance
* **at 35**, she has a 15–20% chance
* **at 45**, she has a 3–5% chance (although most of her eggs will be chromosomally abnormal).

store of eggs (ovarian reserve) slowly declines with increasing age, particularly after the age of 35 in some women. The number of fertilizable eggs has run out long before a woman's last menstrual period. (See ovarian reserve tests, page 101.)

Egg quality A "good egg" is defined by normal chromosomes and, once those chromosomes have combined with those from a sperm cell, the egg's ability to divide efficiently. Older women have older eggs, which may carry chromosome abnormalities, so it may take them longer to get pregnant than younger women. When they do, they are more likely to miscarry and there is a greater risk of chromosome abnormalities (such as Down's syndrome) – 1 in 476 for 25-year-olds, 1 in 192 for 35-year-olds and 1 in 21 for 45-year-olds.

Egg quality declines as a woman gets older, but you can't assess it accurately just by age. Two women of the same age can have different chances of conceiving in any given month. Furthermore, a woman of 45 may have good-quality eggs and still be fertile, while a 25-year-old woman may have poor-quality eggs and be infertile. These are extreme examples, but the point is that, although egg quality declines significantly in the late 30s and even faster in the early 40s, individuals do not always conform to statistics. Your egg quality may be average for your age, or better or worse.

There are screening tests for egg quality but they are far from perfect. Blood tests on days 2–4 of your cycle to check levels of follicle-stimulating hormone (FSH) and the number of antral-follicles (small follicles) are used by infertility specialists to assess your ovarian reserve and your eggs.

Ovulation Ovulation occurs less frequently during the perimenopause – the years leading up to the menopause. As ovulation starts to decrease, a developing follicle does not send a hormonal message to the pituitary gland, which continues to produce FSH and luteinizing hormone (LH) and levels remain high. A pregnancy is therefore less likely as oestrogen levels decline and progesterone production, which only occurs after ovulation, drops off. If you suspect you are perimenopausal, ask your doctor to test your levels of oestrogen, progesterone, FSH and LH. One important question every woman should ask their mother is at what age they went through the menopause, as this can indicate when they will go through it themselves.

What can you do? If you have reached the point where you cannot get pregnant because of reduced egg quality and quantity, you might consider egg donation (see page 183). This would allow you to experience a pregnancy and deliver your own child. There are many social, psychological and emotional issues to consider with this route, however. Whether you try to conceive naturally or by means of assisted reproductive technology, make sure you are as healthy as possible (see chapters 2 and 3).

Vitamins and minerals may improve your chances of achieving a pregnancy. A study by doctors at Leeds University indicated that women can produce better eggs and boost their fertility simply by taking a daily dose of multivitamins and minerals. Researchers studied 215 women undergoing in vitro fertilization and found that women who took a daily multivitamin pill increased their chances of becoming pregnant by as much as 40 per cent. It is impossible to say how many women might be helped by this, but improving your health in this way is well worth doing if you are trying to get pregnant.

Age and male fertility

There is continual replenishment of sperm throughout a man's adult life, so age is not considered to pose such a threat to his fertility. The quality and quantity of sperm, however, do change with advancing age. This is

Signs of reproductive changes in women

Do not hesitate to ask your doctor for advice on potential fertility problems if:

* **you notice changes in the length of your menstrual cycle:** it is either shorter or longer than usual

* **you notice changes in your periods,** such as lighter or heavier bleeding, a different colour or type of bleeding, or spotting between periods or after intercourse

* **you have recently been breastfeeding** and you are still getting leakage from your breasts (and you are concerned about the conception of a second or subsequent baby)

* **you are generally concerned** if you are in your mid-30s or beyond about your natural reproductive potential and/or your chances of success using assisted reproductive techniques should they be necessary.

partly due to a decrease in the number of testosterone-producing cells (leydig cells). As in women, levels of FSH and LH increase, suggesting that men are subject to reproductive failure in old age. There is an increased incidence of chromosomal abnormalities in the sperm of older men (see page 33), leading to an increased risk of birth defects. Sperm development (spermatogenesis) is affected in older men. Sperm count and motility also decrease, and there is an increase in the number of abnormal sperm.

Conditions that become more prevalent in men as they get older may contribute to a decline in sperm production and quality, either as a result of the disease itself (such as diabetes) or of the medications prescribed for it (such as drugs for hypertension). The "male menopause", or andropause, including a decline in fertility, was recently revealed in a study demonstrating that men of 35 and older are 50 per cent less likely, during a 12-month period, to conceive a baby with a similarly fertile female partner than men who are younger than 25.

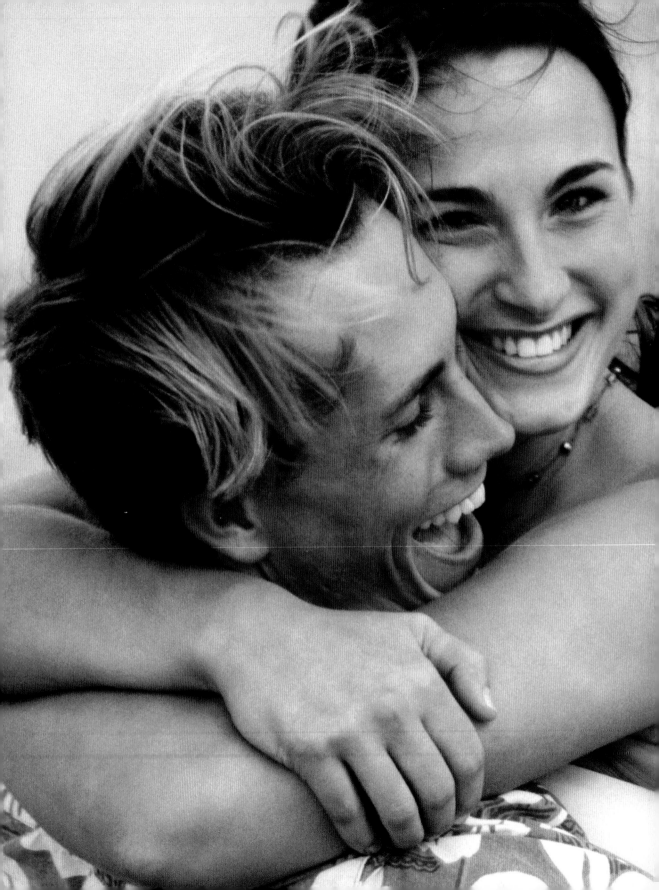

Lifestyle and fertility

When planning a pregnancy, the first thing you need to do is to **evaluate your physical condition** and that of your partner, as these have a big impact on your fertility. By taking stock in this way, you can identify the areas of your life in which you need to make some adjustments in order to improve your chances of **natural conception**. Understanding the importance of the interplay of reproductive hormones and being aware of the **factors affecting fertility** are fundamental. Armed with this information, you can **improve your chances** of getting pregnant.

Planning for a baby

Preparing yourself for a baby is important. You and your partner will need time to work at obtaining the best possible health for conception. You also have to be mentally and physically prepared for postnatal care, then for caring for your baby into the future.

Starting a family

So you've decided that you want a baby. Now's the time for both you and your partner to start taking a good look at your overall health and wellbeing. This is not only to ensure that your body is ready to nurture an unborn child but also to give you the best chance of conceiving successfully.

But being ready physically isn't all of it. You have also got to prepare yourself psychologically. When you begin to plan your family, take some time to consider the following questions that I always ask my clients.

Can you see yourself with a baby in your life? As a practitioner, I feel very pleased when couples reply to this question positively, and describe how they can see themselves with a baby. I believe that it is very important to be able to visualize yourselves as part of a family unit.

Zita's tips

If you've already been trying to conceive for some time, I know that the picture of you and your partner with your own baby may have started to recede as you become more anxious. Don't give up on the dream. Make a plan to review your situation after another six months and in the meantime try to relax and not to put yourselves under pressure.

Have you made space and time in your life for a baby? Many women's lives are filled with work, socializing and a hundred other interests, to the extent that they simply don't have any space left over for a baby. If you and your partner have a gruelling schedule, the chances are that you won't have time for sex; it will also be harder to follow a balanced diet and ensure a healthy lifestyle – all of which is vital to allow yourself a good chance of becoming pregnant. You need to create that space and time in your lives.

Have you made space in your home for a baby? Look around your home and imagine how your baby will fit in and what the baby's room will look like. If the room is cluttered, have a good clear out, creating space in your home for your baby.

Trying when you are older

Increasingly, women are so busy with relationships and developing their careers that the decision to have a baby is left on the back burner until they are well into their 30s. We often wait for that magical point (which hardly ever happens) when everything will be "just right".

Then the biological clock starts ticking. We find the right partner. Work is no longer our sole priority. Suddenly we want a baby – and we want it now. We've all grown used to getting the material things in life as and when we want them. We're accustomed to having control over most areas of our lives – and this includes our fertility. Indeed, up until now we have spent years making sure that we don't get pregnant. We take for granted that having a baby is part of the natural order of things, so it never occurs to us that it may not happen to plan.

Natural conception

But having a baby is not absolutely in your control, and this fact can be very frustrating, especially if you've been trying to get pregnant for a while.

To help maximize your chances of a natural conception, you first need to understand how human fertility works. Many women fail to take into account the possibility that a pregnancy may not necessarily come about just because they have stopped using contraception (see page 47).

Compared with other animals, reproduction in even the most fertile humans is inefficient. Most species ovulate multiple eggs and conceive every time ovulation coincides with sexual activity. Humans have on average a 25 per cent chance of conceiving each month, with most fertile couples achieving a pregnancy within one year. So, with 100 fertile couples, 20 will be pregnant after one month, 16 (20 per cent of 80) after two months, and so on (see chart, below).

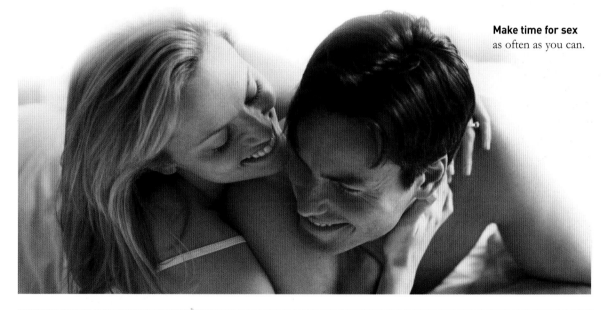

Make time for sex
as often as you can.

Average conception rates in fertile couples

After a year of trying, 93 out of 100 couples (US figures) achieve a pregnancy, at the rates set out below.

MONTH	1	2	3	4	5	6	7	8	9	10	11	12
NUMBER OF COUPLES	100	80	64	51	41	33	26	21	17	14	11	9
NUMBER PREGNANT	20	16	13	10	8	7	5	4	3	3	2	2
NUMBER NOT PREGNANT	80	64	51	41	33	26	21	17	14	11	9	7

Self-assessment

The first step in planning a pregnancy is for you and your partner to get fit and cut out things that undermine fertility. You need to prepare, mentally and emotionally, improve your wellbeing and optimize your chances of a natural conception. If you have already been trying to conceive for some time, I hope the plan I offer in this book will help you find new encouragement.

Taking stock

There are many factors that have an effect on fertility in both men and women, so evaluating your fertility status is a good place to start preparing for conception. The checks here will help you and your partner make that evaluation and decide which factors can be improved. They comprise a list of points to consider that a fertility specialist would raise, and are designed to help you pinpoint any possible problems. On consideration, if you feel you may have a fertility problem, visit your doctor or a specialist for advice and tests (see chapter 4), so you don't waste time. For most people, these checks will help you move towards Plan A (see page 46), making the changes necessary to give you the best chance to get pregnant naturally.

Your fertility check

* **Your age** The older you become, the less fertile you are, so if you are over 35, try to conceive for no longer than six months before having fertility tests (see pages 99–103).

* **Your weight** If you are more than 10 per cent under the weight recommended for your height (see page 29), hormone production may be affected. If you are overweight and find it hard to lose weight, you may have a thyroid problem (see pages 106–107). Ask your doctor for advice and have tests to check for underlying medical conditions.

* **Your contraceptive history** Contraceptive methods you have used in the past may have affected your fertility (see page 47). It may take a while for fertility to return, particularly after long-acting contraceptive methods.

* **Your menstrual history** If your periods are irregular or absent, or if your cycle is shorter than 25 days or longer than 31 days, visit a gynaecologist to have your hormone levels checked. Severe menstrual cramps may be caused by endometriosis (see pages 114–16), which may affect your fertility. Excessive bleeding may indicate fibroids (see pages 117–19). Bleeding or spotting between cycles should be checked as it may indicate a serious medical problem. You may need a smear test: talk to your doctor.

* **Your sexual history** You and your partner need to have regular sex – less than twice a week and you may not be doing it enough to get pregnant. Painful intercourse may be a symptom of endometriosis. If you have been using a lubricant, unless it is sperm-friendly, it may be blocking the movement of sperm to the cervix. If you have had previous sexual partners, you may have been exposed to sexually transmitted infections (STIs – see pages 108–112). Have a swab and blood test taken at a local clinic to rule out STIs.

* **Your general physical condition** Do you have regular smear tests? If not, have one immediately. If you smoke, drink alcohol, take recreational drugs, exercise strenuously more than twice a week, or

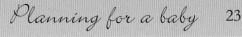

Consult your doctor if you or your partner suspect, after reading these checks, that there may be a problem with your fertility.

don't get regular exercise or adequate sleep, your fertility may be compromised.

✳ **Your family history** Ask your parents about their medical histories to find out if you might have inherited a tendency to low hormone production or genetic problems.

✳ **Previous operations, illnesses and medical conditions** Hormonal imbalances with the thyroid or pituitary glands can affect fertility, as could anaemia (see page 105), gynaecological surgery, cancer or ongoing medication. You need to check with your doctor that you have immunity to rubella.

✳ **Your pregnancy history** A previous pregnancy shows you can conceive, and it's likely you can repeat it. If you've had two or more miscarriages (see pages 122–23), talk to your doctor. Have tests to rule out damage to reproductive organs or infection if you've had a miscarriage, an ectopic pregnancy, a termination with complications or you experience excessive, prolonged bleeding.

Your partner's check

✳ **His age** Male fertility doesn't usually decline until over 50 (see page 17) but reduced sperm counts are more common today. No man should try for a baby for more than six months without a sperm test (see pages 132–37).

✳ **His weight** If your partner is more than 20 per cent under his recommended weight, his hormone production may be affected. Obesity may be linked to other health problems, such as diabetes, which can affect fertility.

✳ **His general physical condition** Ideally your partner should have a physical examination with his doctor, but doctors often don't have the time. If your partner drinks, smokes or takes drugs, encourage him to stop, and to get adequate sleep, relaxation and exercise to promote healthy sperm production. He should avoid extreme diets and taking too much exercise. Wearing tight pants made of man-made fibres during a physical workout or the heat in steam rooms or saunas may impair sperm production.

✳ **History of pregnancies with previous partners** If your partner has previously fathered a child, there is every chance he can do so again if he has had no physical changes due to illness or injury. If a previous partner suffered early miscarriages, he should have his sperm checked for chromosomal defects (see page 137).

✳ **His sexual history** If your partner has had previous sexual partners, he should have tests to rule out STIs.

✳ **His family history** Your partner should ask his parents about their medical histories to see if he has a tendency to abnormal hormone production or genetic problems.

✳ **Previous operations, illnesses and medical conditions** Varicoceles, undescended testicles, mumps, hernia, accidental damage, serious illness or surgery may have affected your partner's fertility (see pages 138–41). He should talk to his doctor if he is worried.

Your state of mind

This is an exciting time in your life and naturally you're keen to do all the "right" things. You may embark on lots of research and make many healthy changes, only to find that you both feel under unnecessary pressure. Always try to relax, be sensitive to each other's feelings, and enjoy plenty of sex!

Making changes

There are many positive changes you can make to improve your fertility, as this book will show. The woman (I find it usually is the woman in a couple) starts the research, reading any literature she can find on the subject (buying books like this one, for example), investing in every vitamin supplement under the sun and embarking on a radical regime that involves changing her lifestyle to incorporate healthy influences and giving up many things she enjoys in life that reduce her fertility. And she expects her partner to do the same, although many men are much more reluctant to do so.

It is important to find out as much as you can about the options open to you and the best ways to get yourself in peak condition for conception and pregnancy. Making sure you and your partner eat a well-balanced diet is, of course, vitally important for all parents-to-be. But I advise moderation. Remember that a little of what you fancy does you good sometimes.

Coping with others

Don't be self-conscious about the changes you make. Couples often worry that friends will notice they have stopped smoking or drinking and draw the obvious conclusions. But these are all things that many people do in the cause of general fitness, so don't worry that they will draw attention to a decision you'd rather remained private for now.

Because you're trying to get pregnant, it follows that you will become acutely aware of other people's bumps and babies. Suddenly they seem to be everywhere. Try not to get fixated on them. You may find yourself having to navigate through a sea of myths, rumours, advice and tips from family and friends, or being hurt by thoughtless remarks and comments. These can be particularly difficult to cope with if you seem to be taking a while to conceive. You know the sort of thing: "He only has to look at me and I fall pregnant", or "You're lucky having all that disposable income and no kids to tie you down".

It may help to have a prepared response for the even worse direct enquiries about when you're going to have a baby or why you haven't got one already. However you decide to deal with tactless enquiries, try not to lose your sense of perspective – or humour. If social events become daunting, don't isolate yourself by avoiding them.

Maintaining a healthy relationship

Dementing your partner by nagging him to make all sorts of changes to lifestyle and eating habits is likely to put a strain on your relationship. Take things one step at a time. At the risk of making generalizations, in my experience men are less than brilliant at taking supplements. I suggest you resist presenting him with a whole health food store of pills and capsules, but instead find one good all-round mineral and multivitamin so that he only has to take one pill each day.

The imperative to start a family is not always the same for the man as for his partner. However ready, willing and supportive your partner may be, the need to conceive rarely assumes the same paramount urgency for him as it does for you, at least in the early stages of trying for a baby. Try your best to accept his point of view and don't pressurize him unduly in any way or let this difference between you cause unnecessary issues and problems in your relationship. It's important that you both remain relaxed, stay patient with each other and keep communicating and sharing your feelings openly. You are, after all, "partners" in this project, as well as being each other's ultimate confidant.

Remember that sex isn't just for making babies and shouldn't be reserved for when you ovulate. Besides, there have been many instances when women have conceived outside of the time during the cycle that is usually regarded as the fertile time. Making love just because you feel like it will be good for your relationship – and your partner's ego.

Forget any deadlines you've set and give yourselves permission occasionally to take time out from trying. Enjoy some passion for its own sake and not as a means to an end.

Relax and have fun! Remember that sex isn't just for making babies. Keep the pleasure and passion fully alive in your relationship.

Your hormones

The proper interactions between hormones are vitally important for the general health of women and men, and for their fertility in particular. Many factors can interfere with and impede these interactions, but you can also influence them – for the better.

A delicate balance

Hormones are chemical messengers, made in special glands or in the brain, that are carried around in the bloodstream to various parts of the body where they have an effect on the functioning of organs and body processes. In the case of the female and male reproductive systems, this means the uterus, ovaries and breasts, and the testes respectively. Each hormone depends on the presence of correct levels of counterpart hormones at a given time in order to carry out its own special role. If the delicate interaction between hormones is adversely affected in any way, then your health may be compromised. If the hormones involved in the reproductive cycle (see pages 10–15) are similarly compromised, your fertility will be affected.

Hormonal imbalance may be triggered by many different causes. An underlying medical condition may affect your hormones, especially if it is a glandular condition such as an under-active thyroid (see pages 106–107). Reproductive dysfunction may, on the other hand, prevent hormones from functioning properly (see pages 113–123).

Dietary and lifestyle factors are common causes of hormonal imbalance. We are increasingly exposed to environmental pollutants that may seriously upset the harmony between and within our body systems. A poor diet may bring about deficiences in the vitamins, minerals and trace elements that have a vitally important role in the production of hormones. Smoking, drinking alcohol excessively and taking recreational drugs further deplete our resources of these precious substances.

Detecting imbalance

You can, however, encourage hormonal balance in the body by following dietary and lifestyle guidelines. First, you have to detect imbalance by recognizing signs and symptoms. If you have suspicions, ask your doctor for a blood test (see box, left), and he will then help you to determine the cause of any problem. If you have a significant imbalance, dietary and lifestyle guidelines will help you only so far. You will need medical help.

Testing hormones

Your doctor can arrange for your hormone levels to be checked with simple tests, usually on the blood.

* **Blood tests** A blood test on days 2–4 of your menstrual cycle can measure levels of most of the reproductive hormones (see pages 99–100). A second blood test after ovulation (on day 21 of a 28-day cycle, for example) can check progesterone levels.

* **Saliva testing** is an alternative method of checking levels of important hormones for reproduction, but it isn't used as frequently. You can take samples yourself at home and then send them to a laboratory for testing. This method needs to be done in conjunction with a doctor who will then be able to prescribe any medication necessary once you have the test results.

Diet and hormones

There are many dietary factors that influence hormonal balance. If you are overweight or eat unhealthily, your fertility may well be compromised. A healthy diet and weight will support all your body's functions, including hormone production and interaction.

You are what you eat

Your hormonal balance and fertility are profoundly affected by what you eat, your nutrient levels and how well your digestion works. Hormone production may be blocked, for example, if you're short of EFAs (essential fatty acids), vitamin A, vitamin B6, zinc, magnesium and antioxidants, resulting in an imbalance that makes conception less likely.

The effects of a poor diet

A well-balanced diet can optimize your fertility status (see pages 54–58). We'd never put second-rate fuel into our cars, because we know it would damage them and they wouldn't perform well. Junk food is second-rate fuel for our bodies. It's low in nutrients and contains additives and preservatives. The body has to expend valuable energy to detoxify itself when subjected to such pollutants. Additives and preservatives can also deplete us of vital nutrients needed for hormone production.

Allergies or intolerances that cause disruption to your digestive function will also allow your body to absorb excess pollutants (see page 28), so it is important to detect allergens and stop consuming them.

Adequate fibre and good liver function (see page 50) are vital as well, because once hormones have carried out their tasks they're taken in the blood to the liver and passed to the digestive tract for elimination. This process cannot be successful if you don't consume enough fibre, or if your liver is overburdened with a poor diet.

Pure, unprocessed food and a well-balanced diet will give your fertility a boost.

Intolerance tests

Wheat and dairy are the most common triggers, perhaps because they form a major part of many people's daily diet. If you suspect that you might suffer from a food intolerance, consider consulting a nutritionist for advice and a comprehensive allergy screening.

SELF-HELP PLAN
The following plan is designed to help you identify which food or foods you might be intolerant to. Cut out all wheat and dairy products from your diet.

Wheat can be replaced with:
* corn pasta, brown rice, rice cakes, oat cakes, rye biscuits, porridge oats, rice flour, millet flakes and whole-grain corn flakes. (Beware of wheat that is hidden as an ingredient in many processed foods.)

Dairy products can be replaced with:
* rice milk, oat milk and tofu. Eat plenty of nuts, seeds and green leafy vegetables.

After two weeks, introduce a lot of wheat at one meal and monitor how you feel over the next few days. Try the same thing with dairy foods (organic where possible).

If you think you have a reaction, cut them out again for three months. If you have no reaction, reintroduce them into your diet slowly but try not to allow levels to creep too high.

Allergies and intolerances

It is worth investigating whether or not you have an allergy or intolerance that may be adversely affecting your digestive functions. If you find you do have a problem and work out how to avoid the substance that triggers it, everything else will start to fall into balance, including your hormone production.

Well-known allergens such as peanuts or shellfish produce an easily identified reaction. But there are other intolerances that can seriously affect your nutritional status, undermine your general health and provoke less specific but debilitating symptoms. Because these symptoms often don't appear for a day or two, their cause can be difficult to detect.

Healthy digestion
A healthy gut wall is permeable, which means that it allows for the transfer of nutrients. Digested fats, proteins, carbohydrates, vitamins, minerals, phyto-nutrients and water are transported across into the bloodstream. A healthy gut won't allow toxins through, but they can get across into the bloodstream if there is a low intake of beneficial minerals, such as calcium, magnesium and zinc, or if alcohol consumption is high. Optimal levels of healthy bacteria in the gut are vital.

Leaky gut syndrome
A weak digestive system and a leaky gut wall can be the result of repeated exposure to allergens. Certain substances (such as allergens or antibiotics) act as a local irritant to the gut wall and make it more porous and "leaky" than it should be. The leakier the gut, the more toxins enter the bloodstream. These pollutants trigger an immune system response, resulting in symptoms such as headache, joint pain, indigestion, flatulence, heart burn, bloating, water retention, mood swings, irritability, food cravings, diarrhoea and constipation.

In a healthy gut, minerals are transported across the gut wall by protein carriers, but these can be damaged easily if the gut wall is leaky. So, the more permeable the gut becomes, the less the body is able to absorb minerals.

So, if you have leaky gut syndrome, no matter how many vitamins and minerals you take, you will not be able to absorb the nutrients you need unless you eliminate allergens from your diet.

Decreased absorption
Other substances that affect the level of minerals your body absorbs include:
* high consumption of alcohol, which destroys B vitamins
* caffeine, which also robs the body of these minerals.
Wheat and dairy are major sources of phytates that bind to calcium, iron and zinc and prevent their absorption. If you are not allergic to them, limit consumption of them.

Weight and hormonal balance

Too many women have an issue with their weight. It's important to be "the right weight", and BMI charts (see below) can be useful, but do not become fixated on them! If you have issues with being over- or underweight, very often there are emotional links to food. Seek help.

You do need to know the implications of weight for fertility. These may make you rethink your target weight, and encourage you to aim for a sensible weight at which you can stay fit and healthy. They may also make you rethink your ideal body shape: research has shown that pear-shaped women are often more fertile.

Being overweight

Excess weight can lead to raised oestrogen levels and prevent ovulation. Fat cells continually release oestrogen, which suppresses the pituitary gland, affecting the release of FSH (follicle-stimulating hormone). Losing a small amount of weight might restore hormonal balance and stimulate ovulation.

Being underweight

Being underweight (by more than 15 per cent) can also stop you ovulating. Too little body fat may cause oestrogen levels to fall and menstruation to be intermittent or even stop altogether. It may also affect the quality of cervical mucus.

Finding the balance

So, if you are underweight, you should gain weight, and if you are overweight, you should lose some. Avoid crash diets at all costs. Follow the dietary and lifestyle guidelines in chapter 3. The detox programme (see pages 50–53) will clear out your liver, helping to redress any hormonal imbalance. I would advise against a radical detox programme if you are trying to conceive, however.

The body mass index (BMI) is used by doctors and nutritionists to gauge your total body fat content. It is calculated by dividing your weight in kilograms by the square of your height in metres. Read the figure for one off against the other on the chart. A BMI of less than 18.5 means you are underweight, while more than 25 suggests that you are overweight.

Body mass index

Weight (stone)	(lb)	(kg)											
24st 4lbs	340	154	71	66	62	58	55	52	49	46	44	41	39
22st 12lbs	320	145	67	62	59	55	52	49	46	43	41	39	37
21st 6lbs	300	136	63	59	55	51	48	46	43	41	39	37	35
20st	280	127	59	55	51	48	45	43	40	38	36	34	32
18st 8lbs	260	118	54	51	48	45	42	40	37	35	33	32	30
17st 2lbs	240	109	50	47	44	41	39	36	34	33	31	29	28
15st 10lbs	220	100	46	43	40	38	36	33	32	30	28	27	25
14st 4lbs	200	90	42	39	37	34	32	30	29	27	26	24	23
12st	180	82	38	35	33	31	29	27	26	24	23	22	21
11st 6lbs	160	73	33	31	29	27	26	24	23	22	21	19	18
10st	140	63	29	27	26	24	23	21	20	19	18	17	16
8st 8lbs	120	54	25	23	22	21	19	18	17	16	15	15	14
7st 2lbs	100	45	21	20	18	17	16	15	14	14	13	12	12
5st 10lbs	80	36	17	16	15	14	13	12	11	11	10	10	9
Height (in)			58	60	62	64	66	68	70	72	74	76	78
(feet)			4'10	5'	5'2	5'4	5'6	5'8	5'10	6'	6'2	6'4	6'6
(cm)			147	152	157	163	168	173	178	183	188	193	198

KEY
- 19 or under, underweight
- 20–24, desirable weight
- 25–29, overweight
- 30–40, obese
- More than 40, severely obese

Hormonal imbalance

A complex interplay of many hormones balance a woman's reproductive cycle. Two important ones are oestrogen in the first part of the cycle and progesterone in the second part (see pages 10–11).

Too little oestrogen

This condition is most common in older women. The perimenopause, the years leading up to menopause, can begin at any time after your mid-30s, and sees a decline in oestrogen and hence ovulation. Ask your mother at what age she had the menopause. Oestrogen deficiency, particularly in the first half of the cycle, may also occur if too much oestrogen is removed from the body as a result of too much wheat fibre in the diet, or if too little oestrogen is recycled via the bowels and liver.

Other causes of deficiency include low body weight – more than 15 per cent below normal – which may cause menstruation to stop and levels of oestrogen to fall; deficiency in vitamin A; excessive amounts of exercise, causing menstruation to cease and oestrogen levels to fall; smoking, which alters the metabolism of oestrogen so that women who smoke are likely to be oestrogen deficient; taking antibiotics, which destroy the healthy bacteria that are present in the gut; and years of taking the contraceptive pill.

Symptoms of oestrogen deficiency include irregular periods, vaginal dryness, painful intercourse, hot flushes and night sweats, bladder infections, dry skin, lethargy and depression and signs of premature ageing, such as memory problems.

Solutions include eating phyto-oestrogens (see box, opposite) or taking low-dose natural oestrogen, available from a qualified herbalist who may also suggest herbal remedies. Para-aminobenzoic acid (PABA) is a component of vitamin B-complex and is involved in the stimulation of the pituitary gland to produce oestrogen. (See page 64 for good food sources of PABA.)

Too little progesterone

Progesterone plays a pivotal role in synchronizing the activity of other hormones. The body uses it to produce three major oestrogens, testosterone and cortisol and aldosterone (stress hormones). It helps to control water balance, it assists in the use of fat for energy, it aids proper thyroid function and is a natural antidepressant.

Progesterone deficiency is the most common example of hormone imbalance in women of all ages, and is linked to ovulation. When ovulation doesn't happen in a cycle, progesterone is at a low level in the luteal phase (see pages 10–11), or production doesn't keep going long enough. This may happen after pill use, a thyroid disorder or breastfeeding. It is known as a luteal phase defect (LPD). Pregnancy is unlikely unless the luteal phase is longer than 10 days. Progesterone maintains a pregnancy in the beginning, so a deficiency may cause miscarriage. You are also more likely to be deficient in progesterone if you have polycystic ovary syndrome (PCOS, see pages 119–21). Progesterone deficiency may also be associated with the faulty secretion of other reproductive hormones such as FSH (follicle-stimulating hormone), LH (luteinizing hormone) or prolactin, and is linked to endometriosis (see pages 114–16) and menstrual cycle irregularities (see pages 126–28).

Symptoms include painful or lumpy breasts, headaches that are linked to your menstrual cycle, anxiety and irritability, sleeping problems, unexplained weight gain, PMS (premenstrual syndrome – see pages 126–28), bleeding between periods and reduced libido.

Solutions might include progesterone therapy (taken orally or in a pessary), which has caused controversy among healthcare professionals. Natural progesterone cream can also be used, but only under supervision. Vitamin and mineral supplements that might help include vitamins B6 and E, magnesium and evening primrose oil. Herbs such as *Vitex agnus castus*, obtainable from a qualified herbalist, can help to regulate progesterone production. Useful lifestyle changes include reducing stress (see pages 40–43), not exercising excessively and increasing low body weight.

Too much oestrogen

Excessive amounts of oestrogen circulating in the blood are increasingly common, not because women's ovaries are making more hormones, but because of greater exposure to environmental oestrogens, found in pesticides, plastics and PCBs – chemical pollutants in water, air and soil. These oestrogens are structurally similar to the body's oestrogen and, although the implications for health are not fully understood, they are believed to mimic its actions, upsetting the balance of oestrogen and progesterone in men and women alike.

Poor diet, with too much refined carbohydrate and saturated animal fat and too little fibre, is also responsible. Saturated fats may stimulate the re-absorption of "old" oestrogens from the bowel. A high-fibre diet helps to prevent this. Eat plenty of fresh fruit, particularly apples and pears, and vegetables, whole grains, oats and oat bran (not wheat bran, which can irritate the intestinal lining). Buy organic produce whenever you can to minimize exposure to hormone-disrupting pesticides, antibiotics and growth promoters. The methods the body uses to expel oestrogens need optimum digestive (especially liver) function, which is compromised by poor diet and a stressful lifestyle.

A high-fat diet is, of course, linked to an increase in obesity which has a disruptive effect on the menstrual cycle. Having too much fatty tissue in the body gives it a greater ability to convert male hormones into oestrogen. Moderate exercise is beneficial to hormone balance as well as weight control.

Symptoms in women include puffiness and bloating, water retention, rapid weight gain,

Phyto-oestrogens

Phyto-oestrogens are natural plant compounds that closely resemble our own oestrogen but are much weaker. They attach themselves to oestrogen receptors on body cells, blocking the effects of both oestrogen and environmental oestrogens, while causing oestrogen-like effects, but weaker ones than those of oestrogen.

A diet rich in phyto-oestrogens can help reduce the heaviness and length of menstrual flow, correct oestrogen/progesterone ratios, lengthen the luteal phase of the cycle and inhibit an oestrogen-dependent carcinogen that causes breast cancer. Phyto-oestrogenic foods are also rich in immunity-enhancing flavonoids, vitamins and minerals, amino acids, essential fats and fibre.

GOOD FOOD SOURCES
Most fruits, vegetables, grains, beans and seeds have a degree of phyto-oestrogenic activity. Particularly good sources include:

* all pulses
* alfalfa sprouts and linseeds (flax seeds)
* oats and hops
* fennel
* parsley, cabbage, Brussels sprouts, broccoli and radicchio
* cherries.

Soya is a rich source of phyto-oestrogens but it may also have mild contraceptive properties. It is not recommended, therefore, for women who wish to become pregnant.

breast tenderness, heavy bleeding, mood swings – causing anxiety, depression and weepiness – sleep problems, migraine, a flushed face, reduced libido, foggy thinking and high levels of copper in the bloodstream. In the longer term, women may develop conditions such as endometriosis or fibroids – associated with the stimulatory effects of oestrogen – gall bladder problems, poor blood-sugar control and an under-active thyroid.

Symptoms in men include hair loss, headaches, bloating, weight gain, prostate enlargement, irritability and breast enlargement.

Solutions include changing to a low-saturated-fat, high-fibre, nutrient-rich diet that will improve hormonal balance, reduce symptoms and optimize conditions generally for becoming pregnant. Other dietary measures include eating live yoghurt containing *Lactobacillus acidophilus* to encourage oestrogen metabolism and the excretion of oestrogen particularly; eating phyto-oestrogens (see box, page 31) to slow down the conversion of androgens into oestrogen and to prevent excess oestrogens from binding to receptor sites; eating vegetables of the cabbage family, which increase the rate at which the liver converts oestrogen into a water-soluble form that can be excreted; increasing protein intake to improve oestrogen metabolism in the liver; and taking vitamin B6 to reduce the effects of oestrogen excess. Taking more exercise will aid the excretion of oestrogens, alleviate stress and help you to lose weight if you need to.

Too many male hormones

Both men and women may suffer from excess androgens, which are the male hormones, in the blood. In women, this condition is usually the result of polycystic ovary syndrome, or PCOS (see pages 119–21). Other causes are poor diet, especially one containing excessive amounts of sugar, refined foods and simple carbohydrates; disorders of the adrenal system; the use of anabolic steroids or corticosteroids; or obesity.

Symptoms include acne, ovarian cysts – which are associated with PCOS – excess body hair, unstable blood-sugar levels, thinning hair on the head, mid-cycle pain and erratic menstruation.

Solutions include a high-fibre diet that's low in saturated fats and refined carbohydrates and high in phyto-oestrogens (see page 31), but you should seek medical help.

The effects of cortisol

High levels of cortisol in both men and women can be associated with stress. Whenever you react to stress, your body responds by producing the adrenal hormone cortisol. This competes for receptor sites with progesterone, making the progesterone less "active" and leading, after a long period of stress, to oestrogen dominance. (Cortisol also increases oestrogen production.) Too much stress will also result in the exhaustion of the adrenal glands and a deficiency of cortisol, which causes hormonal imbalance.

Symptoms of cortisol deficiency include unstable blood-sugar levels and debilitating tiredness. The tiredness is exacerbated by stress or poor diet and manifests itself in two stages. The symptoms of stage one cortisol deficiency include allergies, candidiasis, fatigue and insomnia, premenstrual syndrome (PMS), a loss of libido, susceptibility to viral infections and low blood pressure. Stage two symptoms include alcohol intolerance, chronic fatigue and weak muscles, depression, headaches and unstable blood-sugar levels.

Solutions include reducing your intake of stimulants such as sugar, tobacco, caffeine and alcohol, and making sure that your diet is as healthy as possible (see pages 54–64). Use relaxation techniques to reduce stress levels (see pages 40–43) and then to keep them under control.

Negative influences

Some things are good for you, while others are bad. The good things can help to protect you from the bad, but only so far. In general, avoiding the negative influences that cause damage to living cells will improve your health and fertility.

Making sacrifices

I know that many of you have probably given up things that you enjoy willingly for the sake of conceiving a healthy baby, and that you may feel as though you've been "going without" forever. There is a danger in becoming too obsessive and rigid, and "a little of what you fancy" – the occasional glass of wine, for example – will almost certainly do you no harm. But there are some things you should reduce your exposure to as much as you possibly can.

DNA damage

There are substances and pollutants that you may be exposed to every day, so you should understand the effect they have on your fertility. The substances to avoid are known to cause genetic damage. They are most damaging during the development of the egg, sperm and embryo, and include: tobacco, alcohol at high levels, recreational and medical drugs, dietary mutagens and environmental hazards.

Caffeine

Caffeine is one of the first things I ask clients to give up. The way decaffeinated coffee is processed makes that just as bad as normal coffee. Caffeine robs the body of water and valuable minerals and stimulates the body to produce cortisol (see opposite) which competes for the receptor sites of progesterone, causing deficiency. A moderate to high caffeine intake (more than one cup a day)

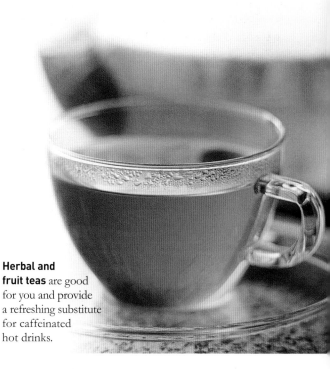

Herbal and fruit teas are good for you and provide a refreshing substitute for caffeinated hot drinks.

can increase the time it takes to conceive by up to 50 per cent. Caffeine is excreted more slowly during the luteal phase (see pages 10–11), which means there will be more circulating in your system during implantation and cell division.

Caffeine increases the risk of miscarriage, low birth weight and pre-eclampsia. There's evidence that if the father has a high coffee intake before conception, the risk of premature birth is increased. So avoid coffee and any soft drink containing caffeine. Tea is not as bad.

Smoking

Smoking robs the body of zinc, selenium and vitamin C, and increases levels of cadmium and lead in the blood. Tobacco smoke contains at least 30 chemicals that can adversely affect fertility. Smoking reduces the rate of cell replication in all organs, so it may do the most damage during the first days and weeks of pregnancy.

Women who smoke are more likely to:
* be infertile
* have lower oestrogen and progesterone levels
* have an inadequate LH (luteinizing hormone) surge causing irregular or no ovulation
* take longer to conceive
* have an increased risk of miscarriage
* bleed during pregnancy
* deliver babies with low birth weight
* have an earlier menopause.

Men who smoke are likely to have:
* decreased sperm density and count
* less motile sperm (see page 136)
* an increase in abnormal sperm
* reduced testosterone
* offspring with congenital abnormalities (because of higher lead concentrations) or a higher risk of developing health problems such as asthma.

These risks increase with the number of cigarettes that are smoked. Also, I've found, anecdotally, that a lot of women going through IVF (in vitro fertilization) who smoke have thinner womb linings.

Alcohol

Many people today think of alcohol as a great de-stresser, and it's easy to get into the habit of a glass or two of something at the end of a hard day. The benefits to your general wellbeing of not drinking any alcohol are considerable, however: you'll sleep better, be more focused, have more energy and feel better all round. If you're trying to conceive, a very

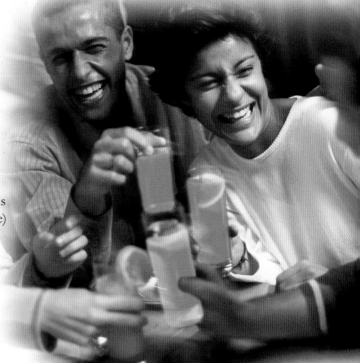

Socializing with friends is a great way to relax – even without alcohol!

occasional glass of wine or the odd beer is unlikely to have a damaging effect, especially if you have it during the first half of your cycle. But give up alcohol completely if you can. Studies have shown that women who drink less than five units (five small glasses of wine) of alcohol a week are twice as likely to conceive within six months than women who drink a larger amount.

Alcohol affects fertility in women by:
* reducing the body's absorption of zinc and vitamin B6. Zinc and B6 are both vital for the proper production of female sex hormones, and low levels of zinc have been overwhelmingly linked to fertility problems
* increasing the excretion of folic acid in the urine – deficiency of folic acid can lead to neural tube defects.

Alcohol is one of the most common causes of male impotence, and 80 per cent of male alcoholics are sterile. It affects male fertility by:

* exposing sperm to the toxic effects of acetaldehyde, a breakdown product of alcohol metabolism
* causing chromosomal abnormalities if consumed around the time that sperm are forming (approximately three months before conception)
* causing atrophy of the tubes that carry semen
* causing a deterioration in sperm concentration and a decrease in sperm output and motility
* adversely affecting the formation of sperm tails
* increasing the production of abnormal sperm cells
* adversely affecting the body's testosterone output, damaging the liver's ability to clear used hormones, allowing female hormones to build up and depress sperm production.

However, these effects are reversible. If your partner gives up alcohol until you have conceived, there will be an improvement in his sperm profile.

Recreational drugs

Cocaine affects the brain chemistry responsible for releasing reproductive hormones. Many couples don't think they have a problem because they do, perhaps, only a couple of lines of coke at the weekend. But *cocaine and babies don't mix*.

Cocaine has a negative influence on fertility by:

* adversely affecting the Fallopian tubes and even causing birth defects
* binding to the sperm, affecting motility and causing problems at fertilization when the sperm tries to penetrate the egg.

Cannabis has an active ingredient called tetrahydrocannabinol that is chemically related to testosterone. It accumulates in the ovaries and testes.

Even if taken in moderate amounts, cannabis can:

* have a toxic effect on the developing egg and disrupt ovulation
* cause a low sperm count, poor sperm motility and an increase in the number of abnormal sperm.

Smoking just one joint lowers testosterone levels and libido for up to 36 hours.

Prescription and non-prescription drugs and herbal remedies

I am always amazed at the number of people who try for a baby while taking over-the-counter or prescribed drugs without realizing the effects they have on fertility. Some are toxic to eggs and sperm. You should be aware of the effects of some commonly prescribed drugs for everyday problems:

* **painkillers** non-steroidal anti-inflammatory drugs (NSAIDs) such as ibuprofen, with heavy use, may interfere with ovulation. Paracetamol is safe.
* **acne relief agents** you should not take Accutane if you are considering a pregnancy. This drug has been linked to foetal abnormalities.
* **antibiotics** make sure you tell your doctor you are trying for a baby if you need antibiotics. Some affect sperm production or motility.
* **antidepressants** all antidepressants can interfere with the hormones involved in the reproductive cycle. Consult your doctor if you are taking these drugs while trying to conceive.
* **antihistamines** these drugs are used in cough and cold preparations to dry up nasal mucus secretions but can have the same effect on cervical mucus. They are also used in sleep-aid products.
* **diuretics** if you experience a dry mouth as a side effect of taking these drugs then they will probably have a drying effect on cervical mucus.
* **expectorants** these are designed to thin bronchial mucus, so making cervical mucus more stretchy, but beware of guaifenesin, which may be toxic.

Drugs to avoid

The following drugs may have an adverse effect on fertility, either on cervical mucus, ovulation or sperm count. Speak to your doctor before taking them.

* antibiotics
* antihistamines
* inhalers
* sleeping pills
* Prozac
* antiviral drugs
* decongestants
* anti-hypertensives
* anti-malaria pills
* painkillers.

* **steroids** drugs such as cortisone and prednisone, used to treat conditions such as asthma and lupus, can, if taken in high doses, prevent the pituitary gland from producing enough of the hormones needed for normal ovulation. However, some women who suffer recurrent miscarriage or IVF failure may be offered steroid treatment.
* **anti-vertigo agents (motion sickness pills)** like diuretics, these drugs tend to dry the mouth and therefore are also likely to affect cervical mucus.
* **anti-malaria pills** these have been linked to abnormalities in embryos. Avoid getting pregnant, or ask your doctor to advise.

Drugs affecting male fertility include those used to treat ulcers or gout, which interfere with sperm production; some antidepressants, which may cause erection difficulties; high doses of steroids, which reduce sperm counts; and beta-blockers, used to control blood pressure, which may cause impotence and decreased sperm counts and motility.

Finally, many drugs affect the way in which the body absorbs nutrients, often causing vitamins and minerals to be excreted. If you or your partner are taking any prescribed drugs, discuss the possibility of drug-nutrient interactions with your doctor.

Herbs to avoid because of their negative effects on fertility include burdock, catnip, cohosh, fennel, juniper, pennyroyal and sage. A study has shown that St John's wort, echinacea and ginkgo biloba may reduce sperm quality and the ability of sperm to penetrate an egg.

Dietary dangers

Dietary mutagens can be caused by "pyrolysis", a process that occurs when foods (especially proteins) are cooked at high temperatures. Pyrolysis adversely affects eggs and the genetic material they contain.

This damaging effect increases if food is cooked in unsaturated fats heated to over 100°C (212°F), as in grilling, barbecuing, frying and roasting. Stick to poaching and braising using olive oil.

Many of the harmful substances produced by this pyrolysis of protein can be destroyed in the digestive tract, especially in the presence of dietary anti-mutagens (see Zita's Tips, page 38). But some mutagens are absorbed and penetrate all the body's systems. Limit your intake of fish, meat, eggs and cheese cooked at temperatures above that of boiling water, but do not eat under-cooked meat or poultry.

Other factors can increase the damage caused by mutagens, including having low nutrient levels of vitamins A, B1, B2, B5, B6, B12, E, folate, vitamin C, the minerals zinc, magnesium, selenium and essential fatty acids. (See Zita's Tips, page 38).

Low protein levels You may be at risk of reduced egg production if your protein levels are low and if you're deficient in individual amino acids. Low protein levels also lead to slow synthesis of DNA and result in a high percentage of embryonic deaths.

In 1989, a study of 200 women representative of all "social classes" found there was a better

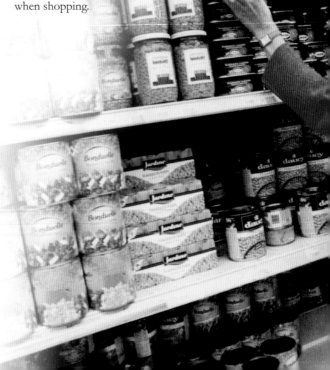

Food flavourings and additives now appear in many pre-prepared foods and drinks. Check labels carefully when shopping.

pregnancy outcome for those women who ate 75g (2.6oz) of protein daily compared with those who ate 63g (2.2oz) daily. Protein intake level was found to be most critical around the time of ovulation. The women consuming 75g (2.6oz) of protein daily from between this time to the end of the first trimester produced babies weighing between 3.5 and 4.5kg (7.5 and 9.5lb) and those eating the lower protein diet produced babies weighing less than 2.5kg (5.5lb).

Flavourings and additives appear in many pre-prepared foods and drinks. Whereas 40 or 50 years ago foods came from obvious sources, many foods today are created from a vast range of chemicals.

Several thousand additives are used in food processing in the UK, but only a small percentage of these ever appear on food labels. Sulphur dioxide

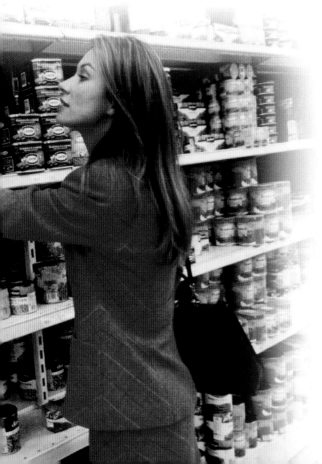

is a preservative that enhances the colour of dried apricots, for example. Even approved "E" additives have not all been fully tested and their effects in combination are unknown. Avoid them if you can.

Salt is necessary, but the amounts added to foods today are very high. I have noticed a direct link between salt intakes and hormonal imbalance.

Aspartame is likely to be found in any sweetener you put in your drink, and it's an ingredient in most foods that are labelled "diet" or "sugar free". When the temperature of aspartame exceeds 30°C (86°F), which it does once it is ingested, the wood alcohol in it converts to formaldehyde (a poison used to preserve body parts) and then to formic acid, which is highly toxic.

Aspartame can have an adverse effect on every stage of the reproductive process and can cause miscarriage by triggering an immune response that could destroy the foetus. Check all labels carefully and especially avoid "diet" drinks.

Monosodium glutamate (MSG) is found in a lot of food from Chinese restaurants and processed Chinese meals. It has been shown to cause infertility in animals. Look out for it also in flavoured crisps, meat seasonings and packaged soups.

Environmental hazards

Nitrous compounds, pesticides, herbicides, fertilizers and environmental oestrogens have all entered the food chain and water supply through industrial farming and as pollutants from factories. Environmental oestrogens may also leach out of plastics such as clingfilm, plastic water bottles and cook-chill food wrappers, particularly if they come into contact with fatty foods.

Every year we each eat approximately 5kg (11lb) of preservatives and additives, and consume one gallon of pesticides and herbicides that have been sprayed on our fruit and vegetables.

Some of this exposure is unavoidable, but eating organic food and drinking filtered or bottled water (from glass bottles) will vastly reduce your intake.

Lead is introduced into our environment through

Zita's tips

There are vitamins, minerals and other nutrients you can eat to help combat the damaging effects caused by pollutants. Most are naturally occurring constituents of plants, including fruits and vegetables. More than a hundred specific elements in foods have been found to be helpful. Particularly effective are:

* **vitamins A, C and E,** which are potent in the digestive tract and continue their action in the blood and around cell membranes. They are antioxidants and help to limit damage by pollutants

* **calcium, magnesium, selenium and zinc,** which are powerful protectors (see page 33) and help to prevent the uptake of aluminium, cadmium, lead and mercury

* **chlorella,** which is considered to be an exceptionally broad spectrum anti-mutagen supplement. A freshwater algae that is a rich source of nutrients, chlorella binds to heavy metals and chemicals that have accumulated in the body

* **coriander,** which is a powerful heavy metal detoxifier as well as pectin-rich foods such as apples, pears and bananas

* **dietary fibre,** particularly from fruit, vegetables, whole grains, oats, oat bran and pulses, which helps in the excretion of toxins from the body. (Wheat bran can irritate the intestinal lining and block mineral absorption.) Soak half a cup of linseeds in juice overnight and add them to food the next day.

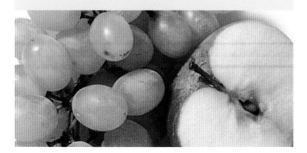

industrial pollution, old water pipes, and vegetables exposed to pollution. Pollutants build up in your body if your intakes of calcium, zinc, iron and manganese are low. Cigarette smoking is believed to increase lead uptake by as much as 25 per cent.

Recent studies have revealed high percentages of lead in some sperm samples. Lead is thought to be responsible for malformed sperm, low sperm counts, poor sperm motility and altered spermatogenesis (sperm production).

Vitamin C may assist with the removal of pollutants from the body, along with pectin, which is found in apples, pears and bananas. You would also be advised to eat foods containing sulphur- and nitrogen-rich amino acids. These include garlic, onions, cooked beans and eggs. Drink 2 litres (3.5 pints) of filtered or still bottled water a day.

Cadmium is linked to increased rates of miscarriage and embryo defects. It accumulates in the body from cigarette smoke, processed foods and some drinking water, as well as from exposure to sewage sludge and high-phosphate fertilizer. It also builds up if you're deficient in vitamins B6, C and D or zinc, manganese, copper, selenium and calcium. Taking zinc in food or supplements (see page 63) can reduce the adverse effects of cadmium.

Mercury is absorbed by the body from pesticides and fungicides, industrial processes and dental fillings. It causes loss of libido and impotence in men, and developmental defects in an embryo if women absorb it. It is extremely toxic during pregnancy and increases allergic sensitivity. Avoid having mercury fillings fitted or removed during pregnancy. Some fish, such as tuna, may contain high levels of mercury and you should limit intake to two portions a week.

Aluminium is easily absorbed by the body and binds with other substances, destroying vitamins and causing long-term mineral loss. High levels of aluminium can lower fertility in both men and women. Major sources of aluminium are saucepans, indigestion tablets, deodorants and anti-perspirants, food additives, tea and also foods that come foil-wrapped.

Copper in high levels in the body is toxic and can reduce male and female fertility. Sources are water pipes, saucepans, jewellery, the pill and the copper coil. Taking zinc in combination with vitamin C can help to detoxify the body of copper.

Bisphenol A (BPA) is a modern synthetic chemical used to make certain plastics and resins. Some research has shown that exposure may harm both male and female fertility.

Phthalates are chemicals that were used in the manufacture of soft plastics and children's toys. They are now banned, but are still found in some make-up products, toiletries and perfumes. They can adversely affect reproduction (as hormone disrupters) so check labels on products carefully.

Additional risks

There are many items used in everyday life that may, perhaps surprisingly, present a degree of risk to your fertility and general health.

Electro-magnetic fields caused by mobile phones may have an affect on fertility, but this has yet to be established. So to be safe, limit your use. Don't use electric blankets: some research suggests that exposure to the current may cause miscarriage.

Tampons interrupt the free flow of blood out of the body, according to Chinese beliefs. If you need to use them on a particular occasion, buy unbleached 100 per cent cotton ones (available from health stores) and, as with all tampons, change them regularly.

Botox is being used by more and more women to delay the evidence of ageing on the face, but we do not know the long-term effects of this on fertility or any other aspect of health.

Flying is a tricky one. I'm often asked about the safety of flying when trying for a baby. I don't like my clients to fly once pregnant as the risk of miscarriage is greater, especially on long-haul flights. But if you're trying for a baby the issue is whether you are pregnant but are unaware of it. Weigh up the odds and don't put your life on hold or miss out on going away unnecessarily.

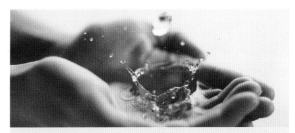

Pollution control

Pollution occurs in so many forms in modern life that it is impossible to avoid it altogether. But there are steps you can take to protect yourself by minimizing exposure and limiting any potential damage to your fertility.

Try taking as many of the precautions listed below as you can. This list may be daunting, but taking any steps you can may improve your chances of conception.

DIETARY
Eat a balanced diet, supplemented by essential vitamins and minerals (see pages 59–64). Wherever possible, buy organic, natural and unprocessed foods. Wash, and peel if necessary, all fruits and vegetables. Avoid processed ham, bacon, preserved meats and smoked foods because they contain nitrous compounds. Avoid canned food – most can-linings contain harmful BPA (bisphenol A). The aluminium in unlined cans leaches into the product. Go on the liver detox programme (see pages 50–53). Avoid copper and aluminium cookware, and aluminium foil. Drink filtered or glass-bottled water: never drink water from the hot tap.

ENVIRONMENTAL
Wash your hands before touching food. Avoid passive smoking. Avoid heavy traffic and close car windows in tunnels. Refuse dental fillings containing mercury. Go outside – natural sunlight helps to eliminate toxic metals from the body and metabolizes desirable minerals. Avoid using any deodorants and anti-perspirants that contain aluminium. Avoid air fresheners, hair sprays, perfumes and shower gels that contain artificial musks or phthalates, because the chemicals they carry affect hormone levels. Avoid chemical cleaning agents and garden pesticides. Do not stand near the microwave oven when it's in use.

Avoiding stress

We're well equipped to deal efficiently with stressful situations, but long-term stress, too often part of 21st-century life, has an adverse effect on health – and therefore fertility.

Stress and the body

Stress is our body's response to a "stressor". It puts us into "defence mode" by sending a message to the pituitary gland, via the hypothalamus, to start the fight-or-flight response. This response:

* activates the adrenal glands to produce adrenaline, cortisol and DHEA (see page 42), which interferes with hormone production
* increases heart rate and blood pressure
* constricts blood vessels (restricting the blood flow necessary for making sperm)
* releases blood sugar to give us the extra energy we need to fight the sabre-tooth tiger or "get-the-hell out", which interferes with hormone production

All this happens in a split second, allowing us to deal with the situation instantly and then return to a state of balance.

Learning to relax is the best way of dealing with stress.

Modern stress

Many of the stresses that people have to deal with today do not involve life-threatening situations. Most of the clients I see, both men and women, are locked into a permanent stress response which they're unable to switch off.

Many are working long hours – 12- to 14-hour days – and coping with stressful situations on a daily basis. They don't have enough time to exercise, eat properly or get sufficient sleep regularly. They drink too much alcohol and rely on nicotine and caffeine to keep them going. They barely have enough time and energy to maintain a relationship and have a regular sex life.

Complex stressors (such as job difficulties, power struggles, rush-hour traffic, money worries, etc.) do not have a simple beginning, middle and end, so the stress response remains switched on and we start to interpret more and more things as being stressful. Over an extended period of time this leads to exhaustion.

It's hardly surprising that under such relentless pressure something has to give, and very often that something is reproduction. Most of the body's energy is devoted to survival, maintenance and essential repairs. In such extreme circumstances, reproduction falls further down the priority list.

The anatomy of stress

Once the body is locked into a prolonged stress response, non-essential functions start to slow down or switch off altogether, as does non-essential chemical production (metabolism). Most of the body's organs and systems are affected:

* excessive cortisol is released, upsetting the body's hormonal balance
* digestion is inhibited
* excess stomach acid is produced
* sex drive decreases
* white blood cells decrease, impairing the immune system, slowing down healing and increasing susceptibility to infection
* blood pressure goes up
* weight is gained
* memory and concentration suffer
* excess adrenaline production leads to dopamine deficiency and depression
* vital nutrients – vitamins B and C, calcium and magnesium – become depleted
* you feel permanently tired.

Blood sugar When you're stressed, the hormones adrenaline and cortisol cause your blood-sugar (glucose) levels to rise so that you have more energy ready for the fight-or-flight response. But then the body produces more insulin to get the sugar out of the blood and into the body's cells, so the blood-sugar level falls abruptly. This is known as hypoglycaemia and a vicious cycle of sugar cravings and tiredness begins.

Twenty per cent of the body's entire intake of glucose fuels the brain – which includes the pituitary gland, responsible for reproductive hormones – so this is one of the first bodily functions to be affected when glucose levels drop.

The implications for fertility

Stress can have a profound effect on fertility. Stress hormones affect the hypothalamus and pituitary glands and reproductive organs. In women, the reproductive hormone prolactin is over-produced and this can interfere with ovulation. The hypothalamus stops secreting GnRH (gonadotrophin-releasing hormone), which in turn will affect the release of LH (luteinizing hormone) and FSH (follicle-stimulating hormone). As these hormones stimulate ovulation, fertility is affected.

Controlling blood sugar

There are many ways to control hypoglycaemia.

EATING SENSIBLY
Avoid stimulants such as tea, coffee, cigarettes, alcohol and sugar. Always eat breakfast. Eat little and often and try to include some protein with every meal. Take a multivitamin and mineral supplement. Snack between meals, but only the right snacks! Nuts, sunflower and pumpkin seeds, rice crackers, crispbreads and oat biscuits with hummus, cottage cheese or guacamole, fresh fruits, bananas with live/bio yoghurt are ideal. Often just a little will be enough to satisfy any cravings you may have.

THINGS TO TRY
Mix protein and carbohydrates in the same meal as this gives a gradual release of glucose into the bloodstream. You will feel fuller for longer and consequently have more energy. Eat complex carbohydrates – brown, dense and grainy with all the vitamins, minerals and fibre retained. Eat fresh fruit and vegetables, either raw in salads or as snacks between meals, or steamed, baked or stir-fried. Add a little unsaturated fat to meals – such as avocado, olives, almonds, peanuts, sunflower seeds, pine nuts and cold-pressed organic olive oil. Dress vegetables and salads in olive oil, lemon juice, black pepper and fresh herbs and seeds. Eat peas and beans – such as kidney, flageolet, cannellini and butter beans. They are a ready-made mixture of protein and carbohydrates. Add them to casseroles, soups and salads.

THINGS TO AVOID
Avoid processed or refined foods – such as sugary cakes, biscuits and sweets, soft drinks, "juice drinks", white bread, rice and pasta. These are quickly digested, causing your blood sugar to rise rapidly, prompting an increase in insulin production. This will cause your blood sugar to then fall quickly, leaving you tired and low in energy, soon craving another sweet "fix". A steady release of energy is needed to maintain your energy levels throughout the day. Always read the labels. Avoid eating fruit after meals as this can sometimes cause bloating in sensitive digestive systems.

Menstruation may become irregular and the luteal phase of the cycle may be disrupted. Semen samples from men under stress show a decrease in volume and greater numbers of sperm with abnormalities.

Stress can also cause a drop in levels of DHEA (dehydroepiandrosterone) which is converted into other hormones. This, together with the cortisol (see page 32) released when you are stressed, may bring about hormonal imbalance such as too high an oestrogen level (see page 31), affecting fertility.

Dealing with stress

If your body is locked into a stress state, you need to address the causes before trying to get rid of the symptoms. Think of it like a paper jam in a printer: even when the paper is removed, the machine won't work because it is still registering a jam. It has to be switched off and on and reset.

Similarly, you need to develop a strategy to help identify and deal with the causes of stress in your life. Write them down, then decide how best to manage them *realistically*. Remember that stress is caused by a reaction to a situation, not the situation itself. Everything depends on how you interpret it and respond to it.

The most common stress factors are:

* work – don't give it up but do try to cut back your hours and perhaps your level of responsibility, or learn to delegate
* your relationship – it's vital to talk to your partner if you are to give and receive mutual support
* failure to conceive – this produces a vicious circle of alternating hope and anxiety. Limit the time you spend thinking about having a baby each day

* coping with fertility treatment – deciding what the next steps should be, how long to continue with it and worrying about the cost. Carry out research and try to remain philosophical, for the sake of your own health and fertility.

Self-help stress relief

There are a number of ways in which you can help yourself feel some release from the stresses and strains of daily life.

Exercise Regular exercise is the best way to relieve stress and improve your general health and sense of wellbeing.

Massage This is a wonderful way of easing tension from the body. Deep massage releases long-held levels of stress and promotes a profound feeling of relaxation.

Deep-breathing techniques Breathing is involuntary but how we breathe reflects our state of mind and emotion. Very few of us breathe deeply enough, especially when we are stressed. When relaxed, we breathe deeply, the lungs fill easily and more oxygen is exchanged. Consciously breathe slowly, deeply and smoothly.

Dao yin is a Chinese system of breathing (and exercise) that helps you to relax, thereby reducing tension and stress, as well as allowing your *qi* (life energy) to circulate more freely, unblocking

Deep massage
soothes away tension.

meridians, balancing yin and yang (see page 72) and charging the kidneys – believed by the Chinese to have an important association with reproduction – with vital energy.

Lie comfortably on the floor and make your breathing soft, slow and continuous. Breathe in through your nose for a count of eight, then out (also through the nose) for a count of eight. Practise this for one week until it becomes natural. Once you've mastered the breathing, focus your mind on the palm of your hand and slowly move your focus along the meridians, finally coming to rest on the conception vessel (see diagram, page 73). Do this exercise for ten minutes every day.

Visualization Some people believe that what you think will happen to you has a powerful effect on what eventually does happen to you. Remind yourself that the body heals and repairs itself and put positive thoughts about health, fertility and conception into your brain. Send thoughts of health and strength to every cell of your body. Refuse to allow negative thoughts into your mind. Positive thoughts will encourage you to do what you have to do, so be an optimist. You will feel better for it.

Transcendental meditation (TM) The physiological effects of TM include a drop in the metabolic rate, which stress revs up. Taking a short course to learn TM can be an investment for life.

Aromatherapy Add drops of an essential oil such as camomile, lavender, neroli, mandarin, rose, ylang-ylang or sandalwood to a base oil used for massage. Diffuse calming vapours around the room with a few drops of essential oil on a light bulb ring or a tissue placed on a hot radiator. A couple of drops in the bath will give you a relaxing soak.

Bach Flower Remedies These are available from most chemists and health shops and may help with stress and emotional problems (see page 147). Add a few drops of an appropriate remedy to water.

Zita's tips

It may sound obvious, but adequate regular sleep is essential if the body is to rest, renew and repair itself. If you have trouble sleeping, try any of the tips below to help you set up positive sleeping habits.

* **Get up at the same time every day,** regardless of how much sleep you have had or what time you went to bed.

* **Try to go to bed at the same time** every evening to get your body into a regular rhythm.

* **Try going to bed half an hour earlier** for a week to see if this makes you feel better.

* **Keep the bedroom quiet and cool,** with an open window, if possible.

* **Keep the bedroom as dark as possible** so the brain registers that it's time to sleep.

* **Keep the bedroom for resting,** sleeping and lovemaking – no phones, computers or piles of papers should distract or disturb you.

* **If you don't fall asleep** within 30 minutes of trying, get up again for a little while. Have a walk around the house, make yourself a warm drink and maybe listen to some soothing music.

* **Limit a daytime nap** to 30 minutes.

* **Take a hot bath with lavender oil** 90 minutes before you go to bed.

* **Try to eat dinner before 7pm** so that your meal is digested by the time you go to bed.

* **Avoid caffeine and alcohol** for at least 5 hours before bedtime.

* **Get some fresh air and exercise** every day.

* **Talk through any problems or fertility issues** with your partner before you go to bed.

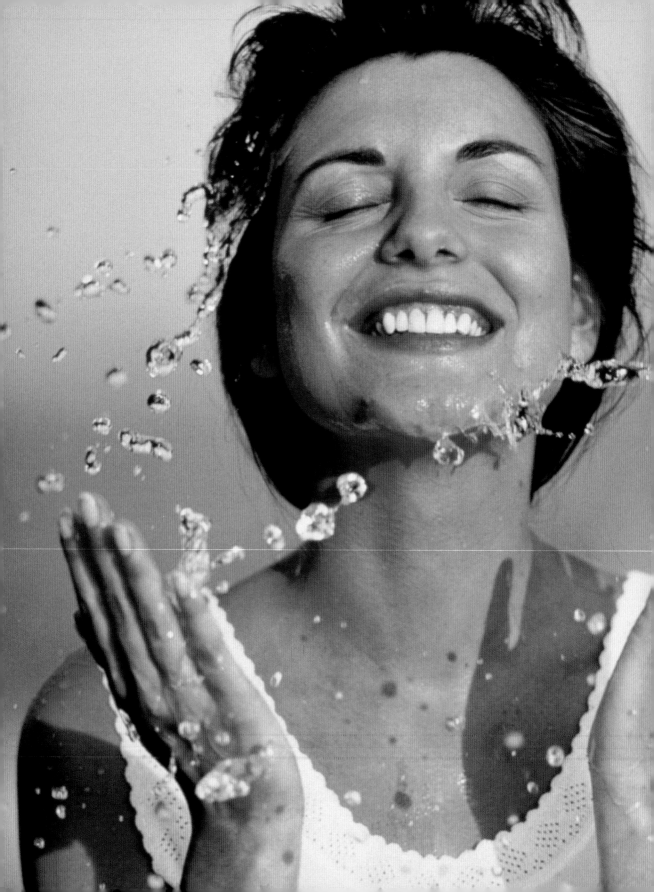

Natural conception

Investing time and energy in *preconceptual care* is a good plan if you want to get pregnant. *Spend at least three months* improving your fertility status by adjusting your diet so that it supplies *essential nutrients to boost fertility,* by taking adequate amounts of exercise, and by managing stress and reducing your exposure to all the things that compromise fertility. You also need to get to know your cycle so that you can identify your fertile time and, during the *countdown to conception,* do everything you can to maximize your chances of conceiving.

Plan A

Now you know how your fertility can be compromised, you will appreciate how lifestyle changes you and your partner make over the coming months will make a difference as you put Plan A – natural conception – into practice.

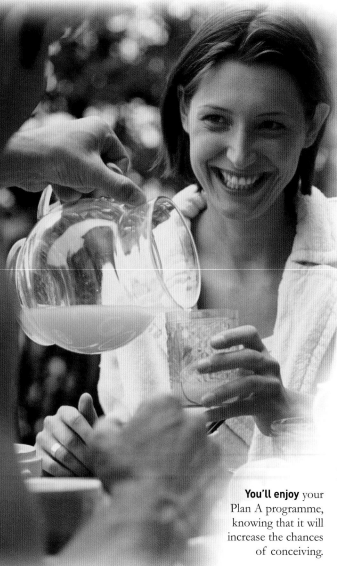

You'll enjoy your Plan A programme, knowing that it will increase the chances of conceiving.

Taking the first steps

You need to consider making lifestyle changes to enhance your fertility status. These will include taking regular exercise (but not too much); following a healthy eating plan, which may include taking nutritional supplements to balance your hormones and get all your body systems functioning as well as possible; and losing or gaining weight if it is necessary.

Work to reduce your stress levels and use complementary therapies to increase your general health and sense of wellbeing. Acupuncture may be of great benefit in this respect and it may also enhance your fertility (see pages 72–73). You might like to consider seeing an acupuncturist regularly while you are trying to conceive.

Research indicates that, if you have been taking the contraceptive pill, you may be very fertile for a while immediately after you stop taking it (see opposite), so don't miss this opportunity to conceive.

Meanwhile, your partner should also get himself in shape. He, too, can start with a healthy eating plan and use the guidelines for physical fitness and a balanced diet that will enhance his general health and particularly sperm production.

It is very exciting starting to try for a baby by looking at and then improving significant areas of your life – physically, nutritionally and emotionally. Understanding your fertility and having frequent sex – and I cannot stress enough the importance of the latter – is a good foundation for successful conception and pregnancy.

Contraception

You may think this is the last thing you need to think about when you're trying for a baby, but it is possible that any invasive methods of contraception you've used in the past may have had an impact on your fertility, so you need to plan accordingly.

The pill

The contraceptive pill works by preventing ovulation, altering the natural balance of oestrogen and progesterone and inhibiting production of LH (luteinizing hormone). Cervical secretions become hostile to sperm and the endometrium becomes too thin for implantation.

The pill contains progestogens (synthetic progesterone) and oestrogens whose molecules are similar to natural hormones, but are present in greater amounts.

One in 200 women finds her periods stop when she comes off the pill; other women, used to having scant 2–3-day bleeds while taking the pill, may find their periods are now heavier.

Recent research now seems to suggest that, with modern contraceptive pills, conception rates are often higher immediately after women stop taking them. Subsequently, the rates dip considerably and do not return to pre-pill levels for as long as 18 months.

Careful vitamin and mineral supplementation will help to correct nutritional imbalances. Follow Plan A (see page 46) for three months while you are still taking the pill in case you become pregnant quickly after stopping it.

Contraceptive injection

This is a hormonal injection given every three months, and is much like the progesterone that a woman produces during the last two weeks of every cycle. Women using contraceptive injections tend to bleed less and suffer less cramping, and, after three or so injections, may stop having periods altogether. It can take from a few months to well over a year – and commonly takes about 12 months – for your periods to return to normal once you have stopped having the injections. Side effects of this form of contraception may include irregular periods, weight gain, depression and premenstrual syndrome (PMS).

Implant

This involves a match-sized rod inserted under the skin that time-releases progesterone to prevent ovulation and also makes your secretions more hostile to sperm. The side effects of an implant can include headaches, weight change, unscheduled bleeding, lighter or no periods, breast tenderness and depression.

Intra-uterine devices

The IUD (intra-uterine device), or coil, is a mechanical device inserted into the uterus. The main action of copper-containing IUDs is to kill sperm (the copper immobilizes them). This is not usually considered a first-line choice of contraception for women at risk of sexually transmitted infections (STIs), although new IUDs with short, single-filament tails have minimal risk of infection ascending into the uterine cavity. There is also a mild risk of cervicitis. If you have used an IUD in the past, it's a good idea to check your nutritional status: look out for mineral imbalance, especially raised copper and lower zinc levels.

Physical fitness

We're well aware of the wide-ranging benefits of physical exercise and yet, with our busy lives, it's all too easy to forget, to let it slip, to put it off until we've finished the other 101 things we need to do. But being fit and keeping active is known to be beneficial for fertility, so it's time to get moving!

The benefits of regular exercise

Incorporating a regular exercise routine into your daily life is vital, but not just for losing weight or shaping the body (although these can be welcome side effects). Regular exercise increases fitness and strength, enabling us to cope with the physical demands of the day and unexpected emergencies. For couples trying to conceive, it oxygenates the body and increases blood flow to supply the reproductive organs with essential oxygen.

Gentle exercise such as walking and cycling tones the muscles without straining the body excessively.

Moderate physical exercise that fits comfortably into your regular schedule, and which you *enjoy*, improves your wellbeing at every level, by:

* boosting the immune system (by raising levels of immunoglobins and white blood cells)
* releasing endorphins (the body's natural painkillers) so that you are less likely to feel depressed and more likely to feel good
* increasing mental speed, efficiency and concentration
* relieving stress
* reducing anxiety
* raising energy levels
* improving self-image and self-esteem
* promoting relaxation and restful sleep
* increasing bone density and mass, helping bones to resist mechanical stress and fracture and reducing the risk of developing osteoporosis
* increasing muscle and reducing excess fat
* stretching and stimulating the muscles and internal organs, keeping the spine and joints supple and maintaining the body's correct alignment to gravity
* increasing insulin sensitivity (so preventing non-insulin-dependent diabetes)
* alleviating the symptoms of PMS (premenstrual syndrome)
* preparing the body for pregnancy: pregnant women who exercise moderately and sensibly suffer far less from constipation, haemorrhoids or morning sickness.

If you're not used to exercising regularly, avoid launching yourself into a gruelling fitness regime. Strenuous exercise more than three times a week can have the opposite effect from what you have in mind and inhibit your chances of conceiving. Instead, find an activity that builds up your fitness levels gradually and, most importantly, one that you'll enjoy and look forward to doing. You'll start to feel the benefits of exercise by doing just 20 minutes three times a week. Swimming, brisk walking and cycling are all perfect.

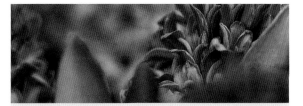

Seasonal exercise

The Chinese adjust exercise to suit the season. Spring, summer and late summer are times of **yang energy** (of warmth, activity, growth and upward, outward motion). Autumn and winter are times of **yin energy** (of cold, rest, reflection, recuperation and downward, inward motion).

SPRING
Spring corresponds to the element of wood and is associated with the tissues and ligaments of the human body. Evenings lengthen, the air is fresh and people emerge from indoors. Gear exercise around stretching, walking and weight training, gently building up muscles.

SUMMER
Summer corresponds to fire and is associated with the heart and circulation. The days are long and the sun is strong. Get as much outdoor and aerobic exercise as possible: swimming, cycling, dancing and jogging.

LATE SUMMER
Late summer corresponds to earth and is associated with digestion and metabolism. It is harvest-time, the sun is hot. Exercise outdoors: try power walking, cycling and swimming.

AUTUMN
Autumn corresponds to metal and is associated with the lungs and colon. Evenings draw in and the frosts arrive. Build up winter strength with qi gong, pilates, stretching and walks.

WINTER
Winter corresponds to water and is associated with the kidneys and bladder. The weather is cold and the days dark. Conserve energy and exercise gently and meditatively with deep breathing, yoga, tai chi and qi gong.

Detoxifying

The liver processes most of the chemicals that enter the body as well as waste produced by the body itself. If this major detoxification organ doesn't function properly, harmful toxins can build up and compromise your health.

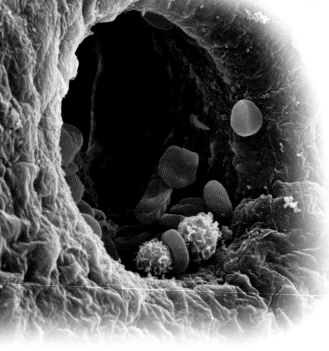

Good liver function

The hormonal balance needed for fertility depends on good liver function. Your liver detoxifies many substances – caffeine, alcohol, drugs, pesticides, herbicides, food additives and preservatives, environmental toxins (from tobacco smoke and petrol fumes, for instance) and toxins produced from bowel bacteria. It chemically alters excess or used hormones ready for recirculation or excretion.

To give your liver health and function a boost, I recommend a liver detoxification programme (see box, below). Many of my clients have found it beneficial. It gives your liver a well-deserved rest since, for either seven or ten days, you don't eat

This section through liver tissue shows a healthy liver capillary (with red and white blood cells). Capillaries supply liver cells with nutrients and oxygen for proper functioning.

The detox programme

The detox programme can be undertaken over a seven- or ten-day period. It is based on two lists of foods (see pages 52–53). "Foods to eat liberally" lists foods that are good for the liver, and "Foods to eat moderately" lists foods that are easy on the liver. On most days you can eat foods from both lists, but for two days of the diet, base your meals solely on the "Foods to eat liberally" list. During this time, eliminate all foods on the "Foods to avoid" list. Eat three meals per day, snack as necessary and drink plenty of water.

10-DAY DETOX
* Days 1–4 and days 7–10: consume foods from either "Foods to eat liberally" or "Foods to eat moderately" lists.
* Days 5–6: consume foods from "Foods to eat liberally" list.

7-DAY DETOX
* Days 1–3, and days 6–7: consume foods from either "Foods to eat liberally" or "Foods to eat moderately" lists.
* Days 4–5: consume foods from "Foods to eat liberally" list.

any foods that make your liver work hard. Instead, you eat foods that are good for the liver, or those that it doesn't have to work too hard to process.

Why detox?

If your liver is constantly burdened, the process of detoxification becomes less efficient. This leads to an increased level of toxins in the bloodstream which can have a negative effect on your metabolic processes. Toxins that your body cannot eliminate build up in the tissues, typically in your fat stores.

How to detox

The detox programme excludes direct sources of toxins such as alcohol and caffeine and also common allergenic foods, such as wheat and dairy, since these can irritate the lining of the gastro-intestinal tract, making it more porous and thereby allowing any circulating toxins to pass across into the blood (see leaky gut syndrome, page 28).

Meat intake is reduced, and fruit and vegetable intake are increased significantly in order to help cleanse the bowel of toxins. This is important because these bowel toxins can be reabsorbed back into the blood, after which they will pass on to the liver for detoxification. The high fibre intake also encourages the body to eliminate toxins that are already present in the body.

Once you start the detox programme, you might experience withdrawal headaches in the first few days, but these usually pass as your body adapts.

Supplements that support the liver

A herb and supplement programme taken during detoxification will give the liver an added boost. These substances are known to help liver function.

Silymarin is a potent liver protective agent. Clinical trials have documented the efficacy of silymarin (an extract of the antioxidant herb milk thistle) for a variety of liver disorders. It helps to protect the liver in people undertaking long-term drug programmes, without interfering with the clinical effects of the drugs.

Detox guidelines

While you are following the liver detoxification programme, in order to maximize its effects and minimize any side effects, bear in mind a few general guidelines:

✳ don't detox if you are on any medication until you've checked with your doctor
✳ stop the programme if you feel pain or discomfort
✳ get plenty of fresh air and, if possible, sunshine
✳ keep warm and get plenty of rest and sleep
✳ don't do any exercise
✳ start the programme at a weekend
✳ consider lymphatic drainage as well (see page 149)
✳ if you have been taking medication, or you smoke, drink alcohol or have a high caffeine intake, drink grapefruit juice with warm water first thing to lessen side effects.

Choline can be bought from health shops in lecithin granules and sprinkled over foods. It is needed to make amino acids, important in liver detoxification. Sulphur-containing amino acids, such as cystine and lysine, are key to liver detoxification.

Lactobacillus acidophilus are beneficial bacteria. They complement this supplement programme by improving the health of the gastro-intestinal tract and reducing toxicity. They are found in live natural yoghurt, but are best taken as a supplement.

Other useful supplements include vitamins C, E and B-complex, betacarotene, the minerals magnesium, selenium, manganese, zinc, copper and molybdenum, and glutathione.

Maintaining liver health

After completing the detox programme, reintroduce allergens (such as wheat and dairy products) one by one. If you don't react adversely, reintroduce them completely, but exclude as many of the items on the "Foods to avoid" list as possible during the preconception period in order to maintain the benefits of the detox programme.

Foods to eat

FOODS TO EAT LIBERALLY

Vegetables – *eat a large variety of vegetables, especially:*

* broccoli, cabbage and cauliflower (all members of the cabbage or brassica family with detoxifying properties)
* garlic and onions (with detoxifying, sulphur-containing compounds)
* asparagus, avocado (containing detoxifying glutathione)
* green leafy vegetables, such as kale and cabbage (containing detoxifying B vitamins)
* artichoke (a natural detoxifier)
* beetroot (another natural detoxifier)
* carrots, sweet potatoes, pumpkin, beetroot, spinach, celery, watercress, peas (all of which contain antioxidants)
* herbs such as parsley and coriander.

Fruit – *again, eat as much variety as possible, especially:*

* apples, pears (core fruits, which contain pectin)
* apricots, peaches, mangos, melons, papayas, pineapples, bananas, kiwi fruits, all berries (containing valuable antioxidants to support the liver)
* lemons – use the juice for salad dressings
* pulses – peas, beans and lentils (for soluble fibre and protein)
* whole grains/cereals – whole-grain rice and millet
* olive oil – for cooking and salad dressings.

Drinks

* fruit (except orange) and vegetable juices – try beetroot, celery, apple and carrot or apple, pear, carrot and ginger
* dandelion "coffee" – three cups daily (a liver cleanser)
* fruit and herbal teas
* juice of half a lemon in warm water 20 minutes before breakfast or on waking.
* water – filtered or bottled only.

FOODS TO EAT MODERATELY

* white meat – chicken, turkey
* white fish – sole, cod, haddock, plaice, skate, herring, sardines, pilchards, tilapia
* eggs
* nuts – almonds, brazil nuts, walnuts
* seeds – sunflower, pumpkin, sesame, linseeds (ground)
* dried fruit – dates, figs, apricots, raisins
* grains – barley, rye, oats
* cow's milk substitutes – oat milk, almond milk
* potatoes
* tomatoes
* live natural organic yoghurt.

FOODS TO AVOID

* non-organic foods
* alcohol
* caffeinated drinks – e.g. coffee, tea, colas (also avoid the decaffeinated alternatives, which still contain substances requiring detoxification by the liver)
* orange juice
* sugar and foods containing lots of sugar – sweets, chocolate (these stress the immune system)
* refined carbohydrates – white versions of foods such as bread, pasta, rice, and also cakes and biscuits
* red meats (these are pro-inflammatory)
* dairy products (these are pro-inflammatory)
* wheat – found in bread, pastry, cakes, biscuits
* foods containing additives and preservatives
* packaged and processed foods, including processed meats
* salt.

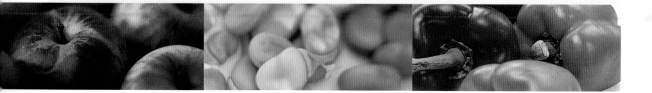

Example menus

DAYS WHEN USING BOTH LISTS

Breakfast

* homemade muesli, e.g. different combinations of oatflakes, barley, millet and rye, with extra oat germ and coconut flakes if desired. Add seeds, such as sunflower, whole or ground pumpkin, ground linseeds and ground sesame seeds. Add a selection of fresh fruit and cinnamon for flavouring, if desired, and serve with oat milk or fruit juice
* porridge oats made with almond milk or oat milk.

Lunch

* grilled organic chicken or poached fish with salad or steamed vegetables, served with whole-grain rice
* vegetable and bean soup with rye bread (make sure no wheat flour has been added)
* jacket potato with hummus
* dessert – fresh fruit salad.

Evening meal

* vegetable stir-fry, e.g. onions, vegetables from the brassica family, red cabbage, yellow/red peppers and carrots, cooked in olive oil and flavoured with garlic and ginger. Serve with whole-grain rice or millet
* chilli casserole topped with live yoghurt
* poached egg on a bed of spinach.

Drinks

* 2 litres (3.5 pints) of water throughout the day, fruit and herb teas, dandelion coffee, vegetable and fruit juices.

Snacks

* seasonal fruits, nuts, seeds, dried fruits.

"FOODS TO EAT LIBERALLY" DAYS

Breakfast

* slice of melon, banana, apple, pear
* poached fruit, such as apples, peaches or plums, topped with sunflower seeds.

Lunch

* salads, e.g. bean salad (kidney beans, chickpeas, green peas), carrot salad (grated carrots, grated apple, thinly sliced red cabbage) and mixed green salad (rocket, lettuce and watercress) with millet. Serve with a dressing of olive oil and lemon
* guacamole with carrot and cucumber crudités
* fresh vegetable soup with beans, lentils and chickpeas
* dessert – a drink of sweet freshly squeezed fruit juices, or fresh fruit salad.

Evening meal

* steamed vegetables or vegetable stir-fry, e.g. mangetout, baby corn, broccoli, kale, onions, garlic, or winter vegetables, e.g. leeks, parsnips, swede, turnip, with garlic. Serve with whole-grain basmati rice
* mixed roasted Mediterranean vegetables served with whole-grain basmati rice
* dessert – a drink of sweet freshly squeezed fruit juices, or fresh fruit salad.

Drinks

* 2 litres (3.5₈ pints) of water throughout the day, fruit and herb teas, dandelion coffee, vegetable and fruit juices.

Snacks

* seasonal fruits, vegetables, e.g. avocado, celery, carrot.

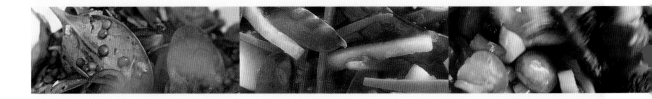

Healthy eating

Once you've followed the detox programme, keep up the good work by adopting sensible eating habits to maintain your long-term health and hormonal balance.

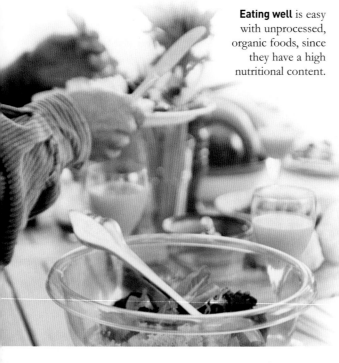

Eating well is easy with unprocessed, organic foods, since they have a high nutritional content.

Most of the nutrients, vitamins and minerals we need should come from the food we eat. But food production has changed. Although there is a huge range of foods available now, most are grown miles away in soil robbed of nutrients by intensive farming, artificial fertilizers and pesticides. Food storage and preservation methods are now so good that we cannot tell how fresh our food really is. Processing, refining and cooking strips away more value. The result is that we no longer receive the correct amount of vitamins and minerals.

Redressing the balance

I want to explain how you can balance your whole system through food. But it's no good my telling you exactly what to eat and what to avoid, especially if you feel you have already given up too many of the things you enjoy. It's easier to change old habits if we understand *why* we should.

Food is not just fuel to give you energy. The quality of the food you eat makes all the difference to how the cells in your body function, including the hormones and cells in your reproductive system.

Try writing down everything you eat and drink over the next few days – you may be surprised at what it reveals. Avoid going on a diet because it has such negative connotations. Just think nutrients instead of calories, and eat the best, the freshest and most wholesome foods you can afford.

Nutritious foods are those that are closer to their natural form – fruits, vegetables, nuts and seeds. Nutritionally inferior foods are generally highly processed and packaged – fast foods, shop-bought cakes, biscuits, pies, crisps and ready-meals.

Nutritional requirements

I don't believe that the "balanced diet" we hear so much about actually exists. For a start, the level of nutrients absorbed from food varies from person to person. Each of us goes through periods of eating well and badly at different times and we each have specific nutritional requirements, depending on lifestyle, metabolism and genetic make-up. Smokers, drinkers, dieters, excessive exercisers or anorexics will all be depleted of certain nutrients, while people who have been on the contraceptive pill or are on medication or daily aspirin will have different requirements again.

Eating well throughout the day

All food is made up of:

* macro-nutrients (proteins, fats and carbohydrates)
* micro-nutrients (vitamins and minerals) and phytochemicals (such as flavonoids, antioxidants and carotenes).

Which of these foods and when we need to eat them is governed by our internal body clock:

* To start the day, we need to eat protein-rich energy foods and carbohydrates together. According to Traditional Chinese Medicine, 7am–9am is the peak time for the stomach, when digestion is at its best, so it's very important to eat breakfast.
* Lunch should be a small, high-protein meal to trigger a rise in dopamine, a chemical found in the brain associated with energy. Eating too many carbohydrates will release serotonin and make you feel sleepy.
* By dinner time the body is anticipating sleep, so eating earlier in the evening will aid digestion. During the night, the stomach empties 50 per cent more slowly than during the day, so it is best to eat your evening meal four hours before bedtime. That way your digestion will be better, you will burn more calories and your sleep will be undisturbed. According to the Chinese, 7pm–9pm is the stomach's rest period.

Proteins

Proteins provide the building blocks of the body. They are needed to:

* repair and renew cells
* transport oxygen and nutrients
* produce hormones
* make antibodies to fight infection
* grow new tissues for muscle, bones and general repairs.

Proteins are made of amino acids and a full supply is essential for egg production (animal studies have shown that inadequate protein intake results in poor-quality eggs) and to produce the hormones FSH (follicle-stimulating hormone) and LH (luteinizing hormone). Cysteine, found in white meat, lentils, beans, nuts and seeds, is a particularly important amino acid.

Both men and women need approximately 60–70g (2.2–2.5oz) of protein a day, making up roughly 20 per cent of our diet. Protein is found in animal products such as meat, fish, eggs and dairy produce and in vegetable sources such as lentils, peas and beans, nuts, brown rice, and sunflower and pumpkin seeds.

The best sources of vegetable protein come from combining pulses and grains, such as lentils and rice for example.

Vegetarians and even "raw food" vegans can have sufficient protein in their diet but they must eat much larger quantities of food. The more amino acids there are in a protein food, the more value it

Protein values

* **Egg** 6g (¼oz) per egg
* **Lean meat, fish, poultry** 25–30g (1–1½oz) per 100g (4oz)
* **Tempeh** 30g (1½oz) per 200g (7oz)
* **Milk** 8–9g (⅜–½oz) per 250ml (half a pint)
* **Yoghurt** 8–10g (⅜–½oz) per 250ml (half a pint)
* **Cream cheese** 2g (⅛oz) per 25g (1oz)
* **Cheddar cheese** 7g (¼oz) per 25g (1oz)
* **Parmesan cheese** 10g (½oz) per 25g (1oz)
* **Cottage cheese** 28g (1oz) per 200g (8oz)
* **Nuts and seeds** 2–3g (⅛–¼oz) per tablespoon
* **Rice, cooked** 5g (¼oz) per 200g (8oz)
* **Cornmeal, cooked** 2g (⅛oz) per 200g (8oz)
* **Bulgur wheat, cooked** 8g (⅜oz) per 200g (8oz)
* **Oatmeal, cooked** 5g (¼oz) per 200g (8oz)
* **Wheat germ, toasted** 8g (⅜oz) per 50g (2oz)
* **Bread** 2–11g (⅛–½oz) per slice (check the label)
* **Adzuki beans, cooked** 17g (¾oz) per 200g (8oz)
* **Kidney beans, cooked** 15g (¾oz) per 200g (8oz)
* **Potato baked with skin, medium-sized** 5g (¼oz)
* **Nutritional yeast, flakes** 4g (¼oz) per heaped tablespoon
* **Most fruits** 1g (1/16oz) per fruit
* **Vegetables** 1–3g (1/16–¼oz) per 100g (4oz)

has as a protein source. Beans and rice are good sources of protein, as long as you eat them in large enough quantities.

In some early research, there was concern about needing to combine proteins so that all essential proteins were available at each meal. Later research has determined that this is not necessary. While all essential a mino acids are needed, they do not have to be eaten together. A "real food" diet with variable protein sources will usually cover all essential amino acids.

Protein in food is slowly released into the bloodstream, allowing for maximum utilization of amino acids. When nutrients are "loaded" into the system, your body must work hard to remove the overload. So, eating protein early in the day and at more than one meal will feed your body best.

Certain kinds of diet seem to come in and out of fashion. There has been a craze to reduce fat and protein (of any kind) and eat mainly carbohydrates, but I do not believe this will lead to long-term health. The body needs wholesome, natural protein and high-quality fats in order to function properly. Contrary to "media nutrition", we do not eat too much wholesome protein. We do, however, eat too many processed fats; processed, preserved and salted proteins; refined carbohydrates; and non-nutritive calories.

If you do not eat fish and red meat you may need to supplement zinc, a component of proteolytic enzymes found in fish, seafood and red meat. Zinc is not only important to protein digestion, it is also key to a healthy immune system, fertility, mood and energy.

High-protein diets (such as the Atkins diet) were once in vogue. Too much protein in the diet, however, may be as problematical as too little. It can lead to excessive levels of ammonia in the body as well as calcium depletion.

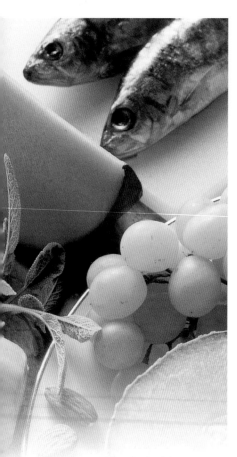

Protein provides the body's building blocks, while slow-releasing carbohydrates give sustained energy.

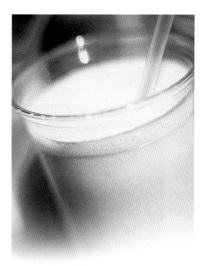

If you enjoy drinking milk, give almond or rice milk a try.

Fats

Fats are vitally important for health and fertility. A range of fats, including saturated, mono- and polyunsaturated fats help to:
* make hormones
* transport cholesterol
* help reduce inflammation.

Deficiency may be manifested as dry skin, cracked lips, PMS and tender breasts.

Sources of fats include butter and margarine, vegetable oils, whole milk and milk products, meats, nuts and seeds.

There are two basic types of fat – saturated and unsaturated.
* Saturated fats are found in meat and dairy products. They go solid at room temperature and are best kept to a minimum since they contribute to heart disease, obesity, high cholesterol levels and an increased risk of some cancers.

* Unsaturated fats are found in olive oil, nuts, seeds and fish. Certain unsaturated fats, known as essential fatty acids and omega-3 oils, are essential for the brain, nervous system, immune system, cardiovascular system and the skin. Some key compounds that are essential for proper hormonal balance are manufactured by the body from omega oils. You should take in more omega-3 than omega-6. Mono- and unsaturated fats should make up approximately 20–25 per cent of the diet. Good sources include linseed oil (made from olive oil), pumpkin seeds, evening primrose oil and oily fish.

Carbohydrates

As the body's basic fuel source, carbohydrates should account for about 55 per cent of the food you eat. They are vitally important as far as fertility is concerned because sufficient amounts of energy are needed for reproduction to be able to take place and to maintain balanced hormones and balanced blood-sugar levels.

Food sources of carbohydrates include whole grains, sugar, syrup, honey, fruits and vegetables.

There are two kinds of carbohydrate:

* "fast-releasing" or simple carbohydrates, such as sugar, refined white flour and processed foods, which tend to give you lots of calories but not many nutrients. You should reduce intakes of these

* "slow-releasing" or complex carbohydrates, such as fruit, vegetables, pulses and whole grains. These are the best carbohydrates because they contain plenty of fibre, give you sustained energy and many contain phyto-oestrogens (see page 31). They can lower blood cholesterol, stabilize blood sugar, regulate bowel movements and give you more stamina. These are the carbohydrates you should focus on.

Micro-nutrients and phytochemicals

Micro-nutrients include essential vitamins and minerals (see pages 59–64) and also plant-based phytochemicals, which include vitally important nutrients such as bioflavonoids, carotenoids, antioxidants and phyto-oestrogens. These are found in unprocessed foods. Eating a minimum of five portions of fruit and vegetables a day should ensure that you get a good supply of these precious

substances, which play an important role in the functioning of all body systems. You cannot have enough of them.

Fibre has great health benefits, including fewer constipation and bowel problems, a reduced risk of breast and colon cancer and a reduction in the incidence or severity of gall stones, diabetes and cardiovascular disease. Eating a minimum of five portions of fruit and vegetables a day should provide you with adequate amounts of fibre. The ideal intake is no less than 35g (1.2oz) a day, although most of us only get about 22g (0.8oz). The best sources are whole grains, vegetables, fruits, nuts, seeds and pulses. Too much wheat fibre in your diet can rob the body of oestrogen. You don't need to sprinkle wheat bran all over your cereal, for example: too much may block the uptake of vital nutrients. Use linseeds instead (see Zita's Tips, page 38) to improve bowel movements, which are important for getting rid of old hormones.

An ideal daily fibre intake of around 35g (1.2oz) has many vital health benefits.

Drinking two litres (3.5 pints) of water a day will help keep your body healthy.

Water is the most important nutrient for the body after oxygen. It makes up 70 per cent of the adult body, 83 per cent of blood, 73 per cent of muscle, 25 per cent of fat and 22 per cent of bone. It is needed for the functioning of every body system, including the elimination of toxins, production of energy, transportation of hormones and development of follicles, and to make sperm, semen, cell membranes and cervical mucus.

Every day, the body loses approximately 1.5 litres (2.6 pints) of water in perspiration, breath and urine. Alcohol, tea and coffee cause us to lose more water and rob us of valuable minerals.

Most of us are dehydrated and don't even realize it, and the consequences can be serious.

* If there is only low-level dehydration, the brain doesn't switch on the thirst mechanism.

* Dehydration increases the production of cholesterol, which surrounds cells to seal in and conserve water, preventing nutrients from entering and toxins from escaping. Taking supplements is a waste of time if you are dehydrated.

* With long-term dehydration, the body rations the available water, diverting it to the essential organs (the brain and heart) and away from the ovaries and the testicles.

To replace lost water, we need to drink at least two litres (3.5 pints) a day. But it takes time to rehydrate. If you pour water onto a plant that has dried out, it will sit on the surface or run down the sides without being absorbed. Our bodies react the same way, so for a week or two it will feel as though the water is running straight through you. Increase your water consumption gradually. Drink filtered or glass-bottled water. Keep a jug of water close to hand at all times, to remind you to drink regularly.

Zita's tips

* **Vitamin D** is important for a number of functions in the body, including fertility and pregnancy. It is classified as a vitamin and a fat-soluble pro-hormone, and new research has shown that many people are deficient in it.

* **Natural sources** of vitamin D are sunlight (the primary source) and food. Low levels of vitamin D are a particular problem in winter when there is less natural exposure to sunlight.

* **Food sources** include eggs and oily fish, such as mackerel.

Also, drink juiced raw fruits and vegetables or fruit and herb teas.

As you begin to rehydrate, the toxins stored in the cells will start to escape into the lymph system. To aid this gentle process of detoxification, go for a deep body massage, have a sauna and take up regular skin brushing.

Balanced eating summary

* Consume fresh food that is in season, and buy organic whenever possible.
* Eat protein regularly.
* Choose good unsaturated fats and avoid "bad" saturated fats.
* Rely on complex carbohydrates for your main source of energy.

* Eat a broad range of different fruits and vegetables.
* Take in sufficient fibre.
* Limit the amount of wheat and dairy in your diet.
* Cut out tea, coffee, alcohol and sugar.
* Drink two litres (3.5 pints) of water daily.

Essential nutrients for conception

Whether it's the many B vitamins, which are vital for hormonal balance, folic acid for developing eggs, or the antioxidizing properties of vitamin C, our intake of a range of important nutrients are essential for good health and especially fertility.

Nutrients for fertility

Although there are many key nutrients for maintaining a healthy body, some play a specific role in enhancing fertility in women. (For key nutrients for male fertility, see pages 76–79.) Your main source should always be food, but modern farming methods have robbed the soil of many vital minerals. Your lifestyle may mean you need extra nutrients, making supplementation advisable.

How supplements help

Taking supplements guarantees you get the nutrients you need. Research has shown that couples who took nutritional supplements over a 14-month period conceived earlier than those taking no supplements. I do not recommend taking vitamins or minerals ad hoc, however. They need to be taken in balance with each other: high doses of one can lead to depletion in another (see page 62). If possible, consult a nutritionist for an analysis of your individual needs and a personal programme to start at least three months before conception.

If you don't consult a nutritionist, take supplements according to the recommended dosages, and ensure that you take them in a way that will maximize absorption and hence their benefits.

Key nutrients for fertility

Amino acids

These perform a vital role in the body and are necessary for egg production. They are found in protein foods (see page 55). There are no RNIs (see page 62).

Vitamin A

This is vital for producing female sex hormones. Food sources include eggs, meat and poultry, whole milk and milk products, dark green leafy vegetables and oily fish.

Vitamin A has antioxidant properties, protects cells against damage and is very important for a developing embryo. There are, however, many concerns about women who are either trying to conceive or who are pregnant taking vitamin A. This is because, in the past, pregnant women have been encouraged to eat liver, which contains vitamin A in the form of retinol. High doses of retinol have been linked to foetal abnormalities. The Food Standards Agency (FSA) now advises those women considering pregnancy against taking vitamin A supplements. An excess can cause birth defects.

▶ **Dosage** RNI women 600mcg/day.

Betacarotene is a plant pigment that is converted to vitamin A in the body. In studies, cows fed diets deficient in betacarotene had delayed ovulation and developed more ovarian cysts. The corpus luteum (see page 10) has the highest concentration of this nutrient in the body. It produces progesterone, so betacarotene may be important for cycle regularity and in early pregnancy. Supplementation is known to reduce the incidence of ovarian cysts. Food sources include peas, broccoli, carrots, spinach and sweet potatoes. There is no RNI for betacarotene.

B vitamins

B vitamins are very important for fertility, especially B6, folate (folic acid is the supplement) and B12.

B vitamins are water-soluble and many are lost in urine. Lifestyle factors such as stress and alcohol, tobacco and antibiotics consumption inhibit absorption. B vitamins are very important for the production and balance of sex hormones. The hypothalamus, which releases sex hormones, is sensitive to severe B vitamin deficiency.

Vitamin B1 (thiamin) In studies of animals, deficiency in B1 prior to mating has been linked to failed ovulation or implantation.

Important food sources of B1 include molasses, brewer's yeast, whole grains, nuts, brown rice, organ and other meats, egg yolks, fish, poultry, pulses and seeds.
▶ **Dosage** RNI women 0.8mg/day.

A huge range of vitamin, mineral and other nutrient supplements are available from health stores and pharmacies.

Vitamin B2 (riboflavin)
Deficiencies in B2 have been linked to miscarriage and low birth weight. The liver uses vitamin B2 to clear away used-up hormones, including oestrogen and progesterone. If these are allowed to accumulate, messages to the hypothalamus and pituitary glands about hormone production may be inhibited and levels fall.

Food sources of B2 are much the same as for B1. The presence of other B vitamins aids absorption.
▶ **Dosage** RNI women 1.1mg/day.

Vitamin B5 (pantothenic acid)
B5 is particularly important at around the time of conception for foetal development.

Food sources include those for B1 plus wheat germ, salmon, sweet potatoes, broccoli, oranges, cashews, pecans and strawberries.
▶ **Dosage** RNI adults 3–7mg/day.

Vitamin B6 Together with zinc, B6 is essential for the formation of female sex hormones and the proper functioning of oestrogen and progesterone. The ovaries respond to deficiency in vitamin B6

by shutting down progesterone production, leading to oestrogen dominance (see page 32). Studies show that supplementation helps to prevent luteal phase defects (LPDs) and encourages the production of progesterone. Research has also shown that if women who have problems conceiving take B6, their fertility improves during a six-month period.

Food sources of B6 include those for B1, plus green leafy vegetables. Zinc aids absorption.
▶ **Dosage** RNI women 1.2mg/day, but I suggest you can take up to 50mg/day.

Vitamin B12 Together with folate, B12 is needed for the synthesis of DNA and RNA. These are important compounds that are part of our genetic blueprint and are involved in the make-up of every cell in the body. Adequate levels of B12 maximize the uptake of folate or folic acid.

The only reliable sources of B12 are animal products, in particular lamb, sardines and salmon. Vegans need to eat fermented foods that contain bacteria, but they are advised to take supplements to ensure adequate intakes of B12. Calcium aids absorption.
▶ **Dosage** RNI women 1.5mcg/day, but I suggest you can take up to 50mcg/day.

Folate The UK Department of Health recommends that women planning a pregnancy should supplement 400mcg of folic acid daily as well as consuming folate-rich foods to reduce the risk of neural-tube defects in a developing embryo. A supplement is best taken for at least three months before you start trying to conceive.

Good food sources of folate are dark-green leafy vegetables, broccoli, organ meats, brewer's yeast, root vegetables, whole grains, oysters, salmon, milk, pulses, asparagus, oatmeal, dried figs and avocados.

Vitamin C aids absorption. It is worth noting that it takes about three months to re-establish adequate folate levels after taking the contraceptive pill.

▶ **Dosage** RNI women 200mcg/day.

Vitamin C

Vitamin C is an antioxidant that blocks the damaging action of free radicals. Too high a dosage (in excess of 1000mg/day) might, however, act as an antihistimine and dry up the cervical mucus.

Good food sources of vitamin C include citrus fruits, rosehips, cherries, sprouted alfalfa seeds, cantaloupe melon, strawberries, broccoli, tomatoes, sweet peppers, blackcurrants, mangos, grapes, kiwi fruit, pineapples, asparagus, peas, potatoes, parsley, watercress and spinach.

▶ **Dosage** RNI women 40mg/day, but I would advise women to increase this to 500mg/day.

Vitamin E

Research on animals has indicated that taking vitamin E along with vitamin C in the treatment of unexplained infertility may improve ovulation. Also, deficiency in vitamin E has been linked to miscarriage in some studies.

Food sources of vitamin E include cold-pressed oils, wheat germ, organ meats, molasses, eggs, sweet potatoes, leafy vegetables, nuts, seeds, whole grains and avocados. A natural (d-alpha-tocopherol), as opposed to synthetic (dl-alpha-tocopherol), supplement of vitamin E is more easily utilized by the body and retained for longer in the body tissues. Check the packet when you buy a supplement to see which it is. Take with selenium and vitamin C for a healthy endometrium.

Vitamin E has anticoagulant properties, so be careful if you are taking aspirin or heparin.

▶ **Dosage** RNI women >3mg/day, but I would recommend 400IUs.

Iron

Low levels of iron can affect fertility (see page 105), and iron deficiency is very common. Adequate amounts of iron help to guard against miscarriage.

Food sources include organ meats, lean meat, eggs, fish, poultry, molasses, cherries, dried fruits, prunes, green leafy vegetables, kelp, spinach, parsley, pumpkin and sunflower seeds, broccoli, oatmeal, sardines and nuts.

Tea, coffee and smoking all inhibit the absorption of iron.

▶ **Dosage** RNI women 14.8mg/day, but I recommend 20mg/day. Only take iron supplements if you are certain that you have a deficiency.

Green leafy vegetables are packed with nutrients, particularly folic acid, vitamin C, B vitamins and iron.

Magnesium

A deficiency in magnesium is associated with female infertility and possibly an increased risk of miscarriage. Animal studies show magnesium deficiency inhibits the use and excretion of vitamin B1. We need magnesium and B1 for energy production: deficiency causes a decrease in the rate of cell metabolism.

The average Western diet tends to be low in magnesium because its common dietary staples – such as fish, meat, milk and most fruits – do not contain the mineral.

Food sources of magnesium are kelp, green leafy vegetables, tofu, pulses, rye, buckwheat, millet, molasses, brown rice, bananas, dried figs and apricots, nuts, barley,

Combining supplements

Most people benefit from taking a good multivitamin and mineral supplement. If you are trying to conceive a baby, specific nutrients may be recommended in addition. You may need advice about how to combine supplements to cater for all your needs.

Identifying needs

Nutrients should ideally come from the food you eat. Ensure that you eat a wide range of nutrient-rich foods. Do not use supplements to compensate for poor nutrition. It is important, however, to take a good vitamin-and-mineral as well as an essential fatty acid (see opposite) supplement.

Depending on the kind of life you lead, you may be deficient in some nutrients. There is evidence that micro-nutrient intakes in the UK and parts of Europe are falling. Those nutrients giving cause for concern include vitamins B2, B6 and C, folate, copper, magnesium, iron, iodine, zinc and selenium. If your lifestyle is stressful or you drink a lot of

The choice of supplements these days can be baffling.

alcohol, it is advisable to supplement vitamin B-complex with some additional zinc and extra vitamins C and E. If you have certain gynaecological conditions, specific nutrients might be recommended in higher amounts (see pages 109–130). In addition, greater amounts of some nutrients are believed to be good for sperm health (see pages 76–79).

Remember that too much of one vitamin or mineral may deplete levels of another, and taking certain medications may deplete your body of vital nutrients.

Official guidelines

Nutrient intakes are recommended in many countries by health departments. In the UK, the Reference Nutrient Intake (RNI) has replaced the Recommended Daily Amount (RDA), although the two are largely interchangeable. The two benchmarks are of little practical use, in fact, and many health experts believe that it would be better to consider the amounts of nutrients necessary to prevent chronic disease rather than aiming merely to prevent overt deficiency.

Dos and don'ts

Don't combine supplements without the advice of a qualified nutritional therapist. Some general guidelines are:

* **fat-soluble vitamins,** such as D and E, should be taken with fats; and water-soluble vitamins, such as B and C, with water

* **certain medications** can rob the body of vital nutrients: antibiotics may reduce vitamin and mineral levels; aspirin may deplete vitamin C levels specifically; vitamin B levels may be reduced by taking antidepressants; and folate can be depleted by contraceptives

* **large intakes of zinc** may interfere with iron and copper absorption (vitamin C enhances iron absorption)

* **iron supplements** may deplete zinc levels

* **taking any B vitamin** will enhance the absorption of other B vitamins, but too much of one may deplete the others

* **coffee and tea** affect absorption of some nutrients.

seafood and whole grains. It is a good idea to supplement magnesium and selenium (see below) together, along with calcium and vitamins B6 and D to aid absorption. Take with protein foods. Alcohol, tea, coffee and smoking inhibit absorption.

▶ **Dosage** RNI women 270mg/day. I would recommend up to 400mg/day.

Selenium

As with magnesium, a deficiency in selenium is associated with female infertility and even an increased risk of miscarriage.

Good food sources of selenium include tuna, herring, brewer's yeast, wheat germ and bran, whole grains and sesame seeds.

▶ **Dosage** RNI women 60mcg/day, but I would recommend 200mcg/day.

Manganese

Studies on animals have shown that manganese deficiency can lead to defective ovulation. It is also believed to inhibit the synthesis of the sex hormones.

Manganese competes with iron for absorption, so food sources of iron should ideally not be eaten with manganese-rich foods, which include whole grains, green leafy vegetables, carrots, broccoli, ginger, pulses, nuts, pineapples, eggs, oats and rye. It is advisable to take manganese supplements with protein foods and also vitamin C. High intakes of zinc may inhibit the absorption of manganese.

▶ **Dosage** RNI women 1.4mg/day, but the upper limit for manganese is 15mg/day.

Zinc

Zinc deficiency is one of the most common nutritional problems that I come across. It is vitally important for growth and proper cell division in a foetus. Zinc is needed for many enzymes to work. Low levels of zinc slow down the metabolism of protein, which is needed for the production of good-quality eggs. Zinc also maintains the menstrual cycle.

Folic acid and iron inhibit the absorption of zinc. In addition, if you drink a lot of alcohol or you have been taking the contraceptive pill, you are more likely to have low zinc levels.

Good food sources include lean meat, fish, seafood, chicken, eggs, pumpkin and sunflower seeds, rye, oats, whole grains, pulses, ginger root, parsley, mushrooms, brewer's yeast and wheat germ.

Vitamins B6 and C may aid absorption: tea, coffee, alcohol and a high fibre intake may inhibit it.

▶ **Dosage** RNI women 7mg/day, but I believe you can take up to 30mg/day, depending on your lifestyle.

Co-enzyme Q10 (CO-Q10)

Co-enzyme Q10 is a fat-soluble substance that is present in every cell in the body, and is important for energy production. Research has indicated that co-Q10 levels tend to be lower in women who have had a recent miscarriage. Supplementing co-enzyme Q10

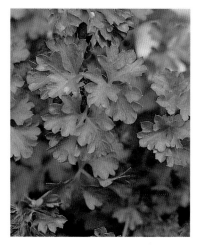

Parsley is a good source of zinc and can be added to many dishes.

may improve fertilization rates in women who are undergoing ICSI treatment (see page 174).

Most of the research into co-Q10 has been done in connection with heart disease and improving blood flow. I therefore encourage women with fertility problems to take it to improve blood flow generally and especially prior to commencing fertility treatment.

It is difficult to obtain sufficient amounts of this nutrient from food sources (although it has been found that vegetarians have higher levels in their bodies). So, supplementation is the only reliable way of increasing your intakes of co-Q10. There is no RNI.

Essential fatty acids

EFAs act as hormone regulators. I cannot stress enough the importance of taking these nutrients as a supplement.

Omega-3 EFAs have a derivative called DHA (docosahexaenoic acid). Eight out of ten women are deficient in DHA. This and the omega-6 derivative, arachidonic acid, are important structural elements of cell membranes. They form body tissue and are essential for brain development in a foetus. DHA is needed for the production of cell membranes in the ovaries.

Women should be supplementing EFAs at least three months before they want to become pregnant, since it takes time for DHA to be incorporated into human tissue. Arachidonic acid must also be present for DHA to be properly synthesized in a baby's system.

Food sources of omega-3 EFAs are linseeds and oily fish, walnuts and green leafy vegetables. Tuna oil is the richest source, but women planning a pregnancy are advised not to eat more than two portions of tuna a week because of the risk of mercury contamination. Supplements are screened for toxins and purified. Fish oils also have anticoagulant properties and may be beneficial if you have had recurrent miscarriages. Be careful, however, if you are taking aspirin or heparin. Food sources of omega-6 EFAs are seeds and their oils. There is no RNI, but 450mg/day is beneficial.

Other key nutrients

There are other important nutrients that are necessary for the maintenance of general good health and wellbeing.

Vitamin B3 (niacin) This is important for energy production and for sex hormones. Good food sources include poultry, fish, lean meats, peanuts, brewer's yeast, milk products and rice bran. B-complex aids absorption: stress, alcohol and antibiotics hinder it.

PABA Based on studies done as long ago as the 1940s, para-aminobenzoic acid (PABA) has been linked to male fertility. This B-complex component may also be of benefit for folate production by intestinal bacteria, the production of red blood cells and the processing of proteins. Food sources of PABA include organ meats, whole grains, brewer's yeast, molasses, spinach and mushrooms. Folic acid and B-complex vitamins aid absorption of PABA, while high stress levels and antibiotics hinder it.

Vitamin K This is essential for blood clotting. Good food sources of vitamin K include green leafy vegetables, egg yolks, safflower oil, molasses and cauliflower.

Calcium This mineral is needed for blood clotting and hormonal balance. Good food sources are milk and its products (but these should be eaten in moderation), green leafy vegetables, shellfish and bony fish, parsley, watercress, spinach, broccoli, cottage cheese, hard cheese, kelp, sesame seeds, linseeds and tofu. Tea, coffee and tobacco all inhibit the absorption of calcium.

Chromium This is needed for the regulation of blood sugar and hormonal balance. Food sources are honey, grapes, raisins, corn oil, clams, whole-grain cereals and brewer's yeast. Supplements should be taken with protein. Vitamin B3 maximizes absorption: tea, coffee and tobacco inhibit it.

Copper This is essential for the production of DNA and RNA (see page 60). Copper deficiency is rare but excess copper can be toxic. Food sources are organ meats, nuts, pulses, molasses and raisins.

Iodine This trace element is needed for the manufacture of thyroid hormones. Food sources are seafood, kelp and iodized salt.

Phosphorus This is the most abundant mineral in the body. It functions alongside calcium. Sources are fish, poultry, meat, eggs, pulses, milk and milk products, nuts and whole-grain cereals.

Potassium This regulates pH levels in the blood. Together with sodium, it maintains fluid balance in the body and transportation of nutrients to all cells. Good food sources of potassium include bananas, avocados, carrots, apples, tomatoes, pineapples, leafy green vegetables, potatoes, dried apricots, peaches, melons, lean meats, whole grains, pulses and sunflower seeds.

Sodium, sulphur and molybdenum These minerals are also needed.

Identifying nutritional deficiencies

As well as maintaining a balanced diet, it's important to pinpoint whether or not you are suffering from any vitamin or mineral deficiencies and to identify toxins that may be stored in your body. You can then take steps to restore the healthy nutritional balance that will improve your wellbeing and fertility.

Testing for nutritional deficiencies

Before you rush out to buy a pile of vitamin, mineral and other nutritional supplements, you need to remember three important things.

* Vitamins and minerals work together in synthesis – they depend on each other to work efficiently.
* Everyone's individual needs are different.
* A good, well-balanced diet that is rich in vitamins, minerals and other essential nutrients will protect and support the workings of your body in the best possible way.

To determine whether, for whatever reason, you are deficient in particular vitamins or minerals, I recommend that you start by visiting a nutritional expert for a full consultation. They will ask you to fill out a very detailed questionnaire about your dietary habits and general lifestyle that will help them to determine where deficiencies might lie. There are alternative methods of detecting either deficiencies or the presence of toxic substances that you might like to consider.

Hair analysis There is debate among health professionals about the use of hair analysis. Many laboratories have produced inconsistent results and reference ranges vary enormously, leaving couples concerned and confused. It is used in forensic science, however, to reveal metal poisoning that does not show up in blood or urine tests. Hair cells are among the fastest-growing cells in the body: as they grow they record all the nutrients and toxins you have been exposed to. Levels of essential nutrients such as magnesium, selenium, manganese or zinc, as well

as toxins such as lead, mercury and aluminium, can be assessed. A supplementation programme can then be worked out. Permed, tinted or highlighted hair does not give accurate readings and, if you swim regularly, algicides in pool water may distort copper readings.

Blood tests The best way of testing your levels of vitamin D (see Zita's Tips, page 58) and omega-3 is a simple blood test. Your test results will determine whether or not you are deficient, and whether you will need to take supplements.

Follow a diet that is rich in fresh, bright vegetables to obtain the range of nutrients you need.

You and your cycle

Getting to know your cycle is the key to understanding your fertility. You need to appreciate what is happening to your body at every stage of the month so that you can interpret signs and work with your natural rhythms to enhance your fertility.

Getting to know your cycle

In my experience, most women take their menstrual cycle completely for granted until they want to conceive. Then they tend to focus solely on ovulation. Ovulation is important, of course, but so is every aspect of the cycle to achieve a pregnancy.

I work very closely with clients to help them understand exactly what is happening at each stage of the month and to recognize physical, hormonal and emotional changes. I'm often astonished at how little women know about the processes of their bodies.

Many women have spent most of their adult lives trying to avoid getting pregnant. They have viewed their monthly bleeds as an inconvenience and barely noticed the parts of the cycle in between. Menstrual flow is a good indicator of general health as well as fertility, but women tend not to discuss the details of their cycle, even with close friends, so they have no idea of "normal" (see below), even though they may complain of feeling "out of sync" if their cycle is irregular. Only when they want to conceive do they become interested in what is happening inside their bodies.

What is normal

What constitutes a "normal" cycle is in fact very hard to describe. Different women have different lengths of cycle and volumes of bleed. What is normal for some women, with regard to amount of blood loss for example, will for others be an indication of hormonal imbalance (see pages 30–32 and 126–30). You should always consult your doctor about any changes to bleeding patterns that you experience.

Western medicine pays little attention to the details of a woman's cycle, but in Traditional Chinese Medicine every detail is considered to be important for diagnostic purposes – the duration, colour, volume and consistency of menstrual flow, as well as physical changes and your emotional feelings throughout the month.

Any cycle lasting between 25 and 35 days is regarded as within the normal range by Western medicine, provided there are no underlying problems. Acupuncture throughout the month can help to regulate a cycle (see pages 72–73).

All the charts in this book, such as the one opposite, are based on a 28-day cycle, which is the average. Yours, of course, may be shorter or longer (see page 81), and this will affect your fertile time.

The perfect balance

Your menstrual cycle is the result of a complex interaction of hormones produced by the ovaries, the hypothalamus and the pituitary gland, which all work together as a unit, sending messages to each other via hormones (see page 10). This interaction affects you in many different ways, from the degree to which you feel sexually attractive to energy levels and mental processing. If you are in perfect balance hormonally, you won't feel the effects of oestrogen and progesterone as their levels fluctuate during your cycle.

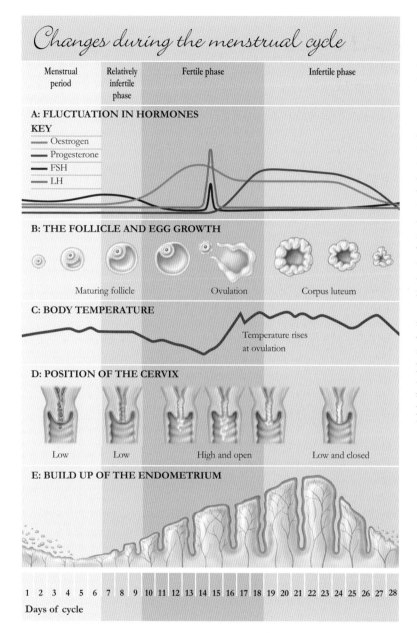

Changes during the menstrual cycle

Menstrual period	Relatively infertile phase	Fertile phase	Infertile phase

A: FLUCTUATION IN HORMONES
KEY
— Oestrogen
— Progesterone
— FSH
— LH

B: THE FOLLICLE AND EGG GROWTH

Maturing follicle   Ovulation   Corpus luteum

C: BODY TEMPERATURE

Temperature rises at ovulation

D: POSITION OF THE CERVIX

Low   Low   High and open   Low and closed

E: BUILD UP OF THE ENDOMETRIUM

1 2 3 4 5 6 7 8 9 10 11 12 13 14 15 16 17 18 19 20 21 22 23 24 25 26 27 28
Days of cycle

Hormonal balance is the key to good fertility (**A**). In the first half of your cycle, the follicular phase, rising levels of FSH (follicle-stimulating hormone) encourage eggs to grow in the ovaries (**B**), which in turn release oestrogen, a signal to reduce FSH. A surge in LH (luteinizing hormone) then triggers ovulation around day 14 or 15. Your temperature rises sharply (**C**) straight after ovulation. At the same time, your cervix is high, soft and open (**D**) and your secretions become "fertile", ready to receive the sperm. In the second half of the cycle, the luteal phase, the ruptured follicle produces progesterone, which halts FSH and LH production and continues the thickening of the endometrium (**E**), or womb lining, so it is ready to receive a fertilized egg.

The timings in the diagram refer to a 28-day cycle. If you have a 25-day cycle, for example, the onset of fertile secretions will be immediately after your period, about day six. If you have a 35-day cycle, ovulation may occur as late as day 21 in your cycle. The consistent part of the cycle is from ovulation to the next period (approximately 14 days).

Most women have some kind of imbalance, however, which means that they feel the effects of hormonal fluctuations. Detecting these effects allows two things to happen. Firstly, it familiarizes you with the workings of your reproductive system so that you can recognize and make the most of your fertile time. Secondly, it identifies imbalance so you can work towards correcting it by means of a programme of detoxifying, healthy eating, vitamin and mineral supplements and complementary therapies (see pages 30–32 and 50–65). If you do have an imbalance, it doesn't mean you won't become pregnant until you correct it. As I said, most women do experience some form of cycle irregularity (see pages 30–32 and 126–28). However, ovulatory problems, which in some cases are caused by hormonal imbalance, are associated with 35 per cent of fertility problems, and it is thought that 10–15 per cent of pregnancies miscarry because of hormonal imbalance. It therefore makes a lot of sense to do whatever you can to correct any imbalances that you detect.

The three-month plan

I suggest you take three months to get to know your cycle, but only if time is on your side. Keep a daily diary, noting every detail, including how you are feeling at each stage, so that you become familiar with your body's rhythms and patterns; you should also begin to recognize any imbalances. If you have already been trying to conceive for some time, you may not feel able to take three months off. Keep a cycle diary anyway: anything you learn may help to improve your chances of conceiving.

The basic process

A cycle begins with the start of your period (fresh red bleeding) on day one. The first half of the cycle lasts about 14 days, assuming you have a 28-day cycle, until ovulation. This is known as the follicular phase (see page 10), and is characterized by increasing oestrogen levels. As you approach ovulation you may experience a feeling of heightened sexuality around the middle of your cycle, when oestrogen is at its peak and you are at your most fertile.

The second half of the cycle, lasting from ovulation to the next period, is known as the luteal phase (see pages 10–11). This is when – if intercourse occurs and all goes well – the released egg is fertilized and starts to implant. If fertilization does not occur, the egg is absorbed and the uterus prepares to shed its lining as a new cycle begins. The luteal phase is associated with rising progesterone levels

and falling oestrogen levels. In the second half of this part of the cycle you may start to experience some of the symptoms of premenstrual syndrome (PMS).

Your fertile time

It is important to be able to interpret your body's fertility signals for yourself. Everybody is different, however. If you're finding it difficult to recognize the signs, I recommend that you see a fertility awareness nurse at a family planning clinic. She will be able to help you understand and chart your cycle.

There are a number of ways in which you can read your body's fertility signs. Although they can all be used individually (and you may find one method that works best for you), it's often easier to use them in conjunction with one another.

Cervical secretions Changes in your cervical secretions are the most reliable indicators of whether or not you are fertile (see pages 70–71). The start of the fertile time is signalled by secretions, so it is vitally important that you are able to recognize how these secretions change throughout your cycle.

Your cervix Oestrogen and progesterone cause subtle changes in the muscle and connective tissue of the cervix. You can learn to recognize these changes by palpating (feeling) the cervix at the same time each day. Your local family planning clinic will tell you how to do this. At peak fertility, the cervix feels high, soft and open. During the rest of the month it feels low, hard and closed. (See diagram D on page 67.)

Body temperature Taking your temperature can be a useful indicator alongside other fertility signs, but don't become obsessive about it. Progesterone causes a rise in your BBT (basal body temperature) of at least 0.2°C (0.4°F) immediately after ovulation. This lasts until the level of progesterone falls at the start of menstruation. Your temperature may rise for other reasons, however, such as viral infections, stress, medication, drinking alcohol or because you've had late nights. Temperature readings that remain on the same level may mean that you are not ovulating. This may happen after using hormonal contraception or if you are suffering from extreme stress.

The LH surge You could use a home ovulation kit to measure the surge of LH (luteinizing hormone) that takes place just before the egg is released from the follicle. Although ovulation kits may identify the two days with the highest chance of pregnancy, you can conceive from sex for five days before ovulation (and the day of ovulation), so if you restrict sex to the limited window identified by the kit you may be having sex too late and not optimising your chances of pregnancy.

Cycle analysis It is important to record details of your menstrual cycle as these will help you to work out your likely fertile time based on previous cycles. Since the fertile time may fluctuate, cervical secretions are the best indicators.

Influences on your cycle

Having a regular cycle that lasts, on average, 28 days will boost your chances of conceiving. Your cycle is profoundly affected by what is going on in your life, from lifestyle choices to which foods you eat.

Light has a surprising influence on your cycle. The influence of the heavens may not be just a matter of the moon's gravitational pull. Sunlight also plays an important role. There is evidence that fertility rates are lower in regions where people spend more time indoors and higher in regions closer to the equator, where daylight hours are longer. Animals that reproduce seasonally move into their fertile cycle when daylight patterns change

with the apparent movement of the sun. This is largely because light stimuli received by the retina in the eyes are translated into hormonal signals by the pineal gland.

Some women with irregular periods have achieved greater regularity by sleeping with a light near their beds, about a metre from the head, for three days around ovulation, and by blacking out their room at night during their period.

Like the oceans, our cycles are closely linked to the phases of the moon.

Improving cervical secretions

Healthy cervical secretions are a key factor in fertility. How hormones affect the feel and appearance of your secretions throughout a cycle can indicate whether sperm could survive the wait for ovulation.

Studying secretions

The cervix is lined with a mucus-secreting membrane. The secretions change in texture, colour and quantity throughout your menstrual cycle. The changes occur because of fluctuations in oestrogen levels. You may notice the following:

* the entrance to the vagina may feel moist, sticky, wet or slippery (leading up to ovulation)
* there may be a residue left on your underwear or on toilet tissue
* the secretions may become very stretchy when tested between your thumb and forefinger (the finger-tip test).

I ask my clients to keep a diary of their secretions, describing them at the same time each day. Most women need three cycles of observation before they are confident about recognizing the changes.

Hormones and secretions

Fluctuating hormone levels cause the changes in your secretions.

* After your period ends, you may have several "dry days" with no detectable secretions. This is the infertile phase: the vagina is a hostile environment for sperm at this time, when acidity rapidly immobilizes and destroys them.
* As oestrogen levels rise as your cycle progresses, you will start to feel moist and sticky and the secretions will be white or creamy-coloured. If you check the stretchiness between your thumb and first finger it will hold its shape but break easily.
* As oestrogen levels continue to rise, the quantity of secretions will increase and it will become thinner, cloudier and stretchier.
* As ovulation approaches, you will have a sensation of wetness and the vagina will feel slippery and wet, with copious amounts of thin, watery, transparent secretions, resembling raw egg white. On finger testing, it will stretch for several centimetres before breaking. These are fertile secretions in which sperm can

Rising oestrogen levels towards ovulation cause subtle changes in the viscosity of your cervical secretions that create an environment in which sperm can thrive. These are fertile secretions.

Cervical secretions chart

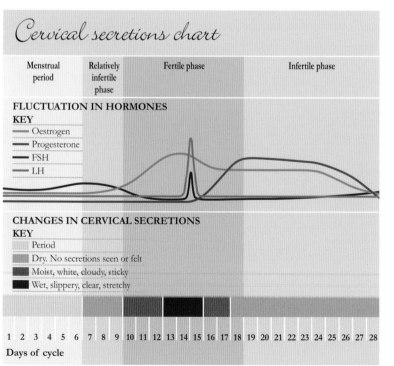

Menstrual period	Relatively infertile phase	Fertile phase	Infertile phase

FLUCTUATION IN HORMONES
KEY
— Oestrogen
— Progesterone
— FSH
— LH

CHANGES IN CERVICAL SECRETIONS
KEY
▓ Period
▓ Dry. No secretions seen or felt
▓ Moist, white, cloudy, sticky
▓ Wet, slippery, clear, stretchy

1 2 3 4 5 6 7 8 9 10 11 12 13 14 15 16 17 18 19 20 21 22 23 24 25 26 27 28
Days of cycle

live – usually for up to 72 hours, but sometimes for much longer. They can now move freely through the cervix. Under a microscope, you would see the long channels along which the sperm swim. Only normal sperm can fit into these channels. Women often worry about sperm leaking out after intercourse, but if fertile secretions are present, sperm will swim through it.

* The peak day for fertile secretions (directly prior to ovulation) is the last day, when the secretions exhibit their most fertile characteristics. After this, you will quickly feel dry or sticky again. Thicker cervical secretions, caused by a rise in progesterone, form a plug at the cervix which serves as an impenetrable barrier.

Problems with secretions

If you are having problems finding fertile secretions, you may be ovulating early in your cycle, at the end of a period, so it is mixed up with menstrual blood.

The cervix responds to increased oestrogen levels by opening the glands in the cervical canal to release cervical secretions. Insufficient secretions may indicate low oestrogen levels (see page 30), which is a condition most common in older women during the perimenopause and menopause.

Other causes for inadequate secretions are:

* low body weight (with a low BMI – see page 29), which can cause oestrogen levels to fall and periods to stop
* rapid change in weight, which may suppress ovulation
* prescribed drugs whose side effect is to dry out, thicken or decrease amounts of secretions: these include antihistamines, cimetidine (for peptic ulcers) and clomiphene (for ovulation)
* too much exercise, which reduces circulating oestrogens
* smoking, which alters the metabolism of oestrogen
* high doses of vitamin C (>3g), which may dry up secretions
* perfumed toilet paper, fabric softener and tampons, which may distort cervical secretions
* vaginal lubricants, which may restrict the movement of sperm
* an incorrect pH balance – highly acidic secretions are hostile to sperm (see box, right)
* poor sex technique – if you are not producing arousal fluid, sex will be more difficult.

Improving secretions

Drinking plenty of water can help to increase the volume and health of your cervical secretions.

There have been suggestions that using egg white (if you are not allergic to eggs) or saliva, or drinking cough mixture, will improve cervical secretions, but there is not enough research to validate these claims.

Foods for PH balance

Sperm prefer alkaline conditions. Although there is no conclusive research, eating more alkaline foods and fewer acidic foods may help to improve the pH balance of secretions.

HIGH ALKALINE
Millet, almonds, seaweed, beets, artichokes, asparagus, greens, broccoli, Brussels sprouts, celery, cabbage, carrots, cauliflower, kale, cucumber, endive, escarole, leeks, kohlrabi, lettuce, onions, garlic, ginger, parsley, potatoes, sweet potatoes, pumpkins, turnips, watercress.

ALKALINE
Brown rice, apples, apricots, fresh figs, bananas, berries, melons, kiwi fruit, grapes, lemons, limes, pears, plums, peaches, mangos, papayas, bamboo shoots, bok choy, parsnips, aubergines, okra, peppers, radishes, Swiss chard, rhubarb, spinach.

NEUTRAL
Yoghurt, butter.

LOW ACID
Lamb, chicken, turkey, goose, duck, salmon, white fish, eggs, beans, barley, buckwheat, oats, rye, white rice, mushrooms, raisins.

HIGH ACID
Beef, veal, pork, ham, bacon, cheese, goat's and cow's milk, wheat, corn.

Acupuncture

Although my fertility practice is grounded in Western medicine, I frequently use acupuncture to regulate the menstrual cycle or to treat other fertility problems.

Traditional Chinese Medicine (TCM)
According to ancient Chinese beliefs, we all have a vital life force or energy known as *qi* (pronounced chee), which flows along invisible pathways called meridians (see opposite). Most of the principal meridians are named after the major internal organs through which they pass. The Conception Vessel runs up the middle of the body and has important acupoints associated with it.

Each organ plays a role in maintaining a smooth flow of *qi*, which in turn allows body systems to function well. Treatment is given to support a weak organ and restore balance. Most people have a constitutional weakness that affects their flow of *qi*. Symptoms of illness indicate imbalance in the meridian of one organ or another. Each organ exhibits a characteristic pattern of disharmony that a trained practitioner can identify from symptoms.

The meridians associated with reproduction are the kidneys, spleen and liver. If symptoms suggest a "kidney deficiency", for example, acupuncture on specific acupoints along that meridian will support the kidneys and restore balance. According to the Chinese, the kidneys store reproductive *jing* (see below) or essence. Good *jing* means strong sperm, strong eggs, and strong and healthy children. Many women I see have a kidney deficiency, their kidney energy depleted by previous pregnancies, recurrent miscarriage or IVF treatment. It doesn't mean there is something wrong with your kidneys.

In order to re-establish balance in a woman's body and enhance her fertility, I treat her on a weekly basis. In Chinese medicine blood flow is considered very important, and acupoints may be used to relieve menstrual pain, encourage healthy blood flow, replenish energy by "building" the blood, boost ovulation and encourage implantation.

Yin and yang
As well as *qi*, the Chinese believe in the opposing forces of *yin* and *yang*. These make up the two complementary halves of a whole, and each represents the opposite of the other in everything.

Acupoints
Acupoints, or acupuncture points – 365 of them in all – are located along the meridians. Acupoints resemble tiny valves through which the flow of *qi* can be regulated. Certain points are particularly

Acupuncture and fertility

Research has shown that acupuncture may help to relieve the symptoms of many conditions, some of which may compromise fertility. These ailments include dysmenorrhoea (painful periods), amenorrhoea (no periods) and other menstrual cycle irregularities and reproduction system problems, including PMS (premenstrual syndrome), hormonal imbalance, anovulation (no ovulation), endometriosis, breast pain, prostate pain, urinary and bladder pain and menopause.

A lot of the research has been done on the use of auricular (ear) acupuncture and electro-acupuncture. It is my belief that it is also of benefit during in vitro fertilization (IVF). (See page 163.)

relevant for fertility, as their names suggest, such as Door of Infants and the Gate of Life. To find an acupoint, a practitioner will palpate along the relevant meridian until he or she locates a little dip. As the fine needle is inserted, you will probably experience a dull sensation.

Diagnosis and treatment

The ancient Chinese did not have scans and blood tests for diagnosis, but instead looked to natural laws and cycles and the ways in which they are reflected in people to identify imbalances. Many details about an individual are important in diagnosis: the sound of the voice, skin tone, body odour, preferred season, food likes and dislikes, dominant emotions and sleep patterns.

The tongue is an important diagnostic tool. Each area of the tongue represents a different part of the body: I look for colour, coating and the presence of any cracks to aid diagnosis.

Abdominal diagnosis is all about temperature. If *qi* is flowing smoothly, your temperature should be even all over. The Chinese believe that you cannot "grow" a baby in an abdomen that is cold, but many of my female clients come to me with a lower abdomen that feels cold to the touch.

The Chinese see the ear as a representation of an inverted foetus. All the major meridians cross the ear and it has more than 120 acupoints. It is particularly useful for treating hormonal imbalance.

Finally, pulse diagnosis recognizes six pulses on the hand, each relating to specific organs. The quality of a pulse varies throughout a woman's cycle and imbalances can be detected from these changes. Reading the pulses forms a crucial part of diagnosis.

Electro-acupuncture makes use of a machine to boost the treatment. It is particularly useful for relieving pain, boosting ovulation and regulating the menstrual cycle.

Acupuncture for you

Acupuncture may improve your general health, alleviate underlying conditions preventing

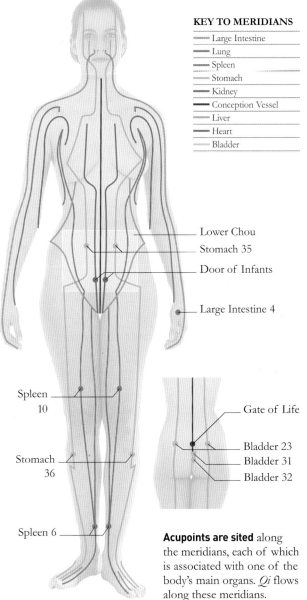

KEY TO MERIDIANS
— Large Intestine
— Lung
— Spleen
— Stomach
— Kidney
— Conception Vessel
— Liver
— Heart
— Bladder

Lower Chou
Stomach 35
Door of Infants

Large Intestine 4

Spleen 10

Stomach 36

Spleen 6

Gate of Life

Bladder 23
Bladder 31
Bladder 32

Acupoints are sited along the meridians, each of which is associated with one of the body's main organs. *Qi* flows along these meridians.

conception or enhance the efficacy of fertility treatments. Find a practitioner who specializes in fertility, especially if you are older or you have a reproductive dysfunction. Be prepared to change many aspects of your life in order to support treatment: exercise, diet and stress management for example. Chinese medicine treats the whole person at a physical and mental/emotional level.

Improving sperm quality

It may be difficult to get your partner to work at improving his sperm quality unless he knows there is a problem, but his general health will also be improved by a few simple measures.

100 days to healthy sperm

By making a few simple changes to his diet and lifestyle, your partner can make a significant difference to the quality and quantity of his sperm. But improvements don't happen overnight. It takes 100 days for sperm to develop – 74 days to form and 20–30 days to mature completely. So a programme to improve sperm quality and count should begin at least 100 days before conception.

What constitutes good sperm?

Three essential factors are involved:
* sperm count – the average count should be more than 20 million sperm per millilitre of ejaculate
* morphology – this is the shape of the sperm
* motility – how fast sperm swim and how they progress forwards.

In general, the higher the count, the higher the percentage of normal sperm and motile sperm, therefore the greater the chance of conception.

Lifestyle changes

Your partner should try to incorporate the following changes into his daily life for the next three months or so. By then, he will more than likely have improved his sperm quality (depending on why it was low in the first place), and his general health and fitness levels will be much improved. He will find he has higher energy levels, more efficient digestion, fewer headaches and more restful sleep.

Encourage your partner to:
* eat healthily and take a good multivitamin and mineral and DHA supplements (see pages 76–79)

Moderate exercise can help improve his sperm count, but excessive workouts could reduce it.

* go on the detox programme for seven or ten days (see pages 50–53) to improve his liver function and hormonal balance
* find some time every day to unwind and let go of stress – he may consider learning deep breathing techniques or meditation (see pages 42–43)
* have a weekly acupuncture treatment (on the kidney meridian) for general health and energy levels if problems are detected
* exercise and be active – taking the stairs instead of the lift or parking further away from his destination and walking – all these measures will improve his general fitness and reduce stress levels. But he must not overdo things, as prolonged vigorous exercise more than three times a week should be avoided
* stop smoking, cut down on alcohol, avoid recreational drugs and reduce his caffeine intake
* drink at least 2 litres (3.5 pints) of water a day – semen is made up largely of water.

Negative influences on sperm formation

In order to give himself the best chance of producing fertile sperm, your partner should try to avoid the following negative influences.

High temperatures

Sperm cells will not develop or function well if their temperature is higher than 32°C (90°F), despite the body's normal core temperature being 37°C (98.6°F). In fact, spending a long time in a hot bath, sauna or Jacuzzi can "cook" sperm cells. Long-distance driving also heats the scrotum.

Wearing athletic supports or tight-fitting underwear made from synthetic fibres can also reduce sperm count. If your partner wears loose-fitting, cotton boxer shorts and avoids spending too long in high temperatures, sperm recovery will take only 100 days.

Stress

Long hours, poor diet and high levels of stress take their toll on sperm production. Constant stress results in the body fighting on all fronts to get blood to the heart, lungs and brain. Forget below-the-waist activity: energy is needed to make sperm and if it is diverted to other parts of the body, sperm production suffers. Both of you should take time to relax each day.

Alcohol

Alcohol has many negative effects on male fertility, including interfering with the secretion of testosterone, speeding up its conversion to oestrogen, lowering sperm count and reducing sex drive (see also page 34). The breakdown product of alcohol metabolism, acetaldehyde, is toxic to sperm and also causes free radical damage. Damage is not permanent if your partner stops drinking now.

Smoking

Smoking doubles the number of free radicals produced in the body every second, reduces sperm count and sperm motility, and increases the risk of sperm abnormalities and genetic defects in the embryo. Your partner should stop now.

Drugs

The active ingredient in cannabis is chemically related to testosterone. It tends to build up in the testicles, lowering libido and causing impotence. Cannabis lowers sperm count, as does cocaine.

A number of prescribed drugs can also have detrimental effects on sperm (see pages 35–36).

Antioxidants

Around 40 per cent of sperm damage is thought to be caused by oxidizing free radicals. Antioxidants vitamins C and E, betacarotene, selenium and zinc help to protect sperm from damage, preventing them from clumping together, increasing motility and reducing the risk of genetic abnormalities in any offspring produced from them.

Foods that are high in antioxidants include blackberries, blueberries, garlic, kale, strawberries, Brussels sprouts, plums, alfalfa sprouts, broccoli and red peppers.

Caffeine

Caffeine may impair sperm production, cause chromosomal abnormalities and affect sperm motility (see also page 33).

Medical problems

A hernia repair, tubule infection, chlamydia or mumps can affect sperm count. Underlying illnesses such as diabetes may affect sperm production. An acidophilus supplement will replace depleted beneficial bacteria in the gut following the use of antibiotics.

Exercise

Exercise is important for good health, but excessive amounts of punishing exercise, such as long-distance running, may lower sperm count and reduce testosterone production temporarily.

Toxins and pollutants

Toxins and pollutants, including pesticides and heavy metals, are very harmful to sperm production (see pages 37–39). Encourage your partner to include organic products in his diet as much as possible. Many men face occupational hazards in the form of X-rays, solvents, paint products and toxic metals (see also pages 37–39).

Environmental oestrogens

We all take in far more oestrogens than 50 years ago, leading to hormonal imbalances in both men and women (see page 31). There are traces of oestrogen drugs in drinking water, for example, and livestock are given increasing amounts of growth hormones.

Diet and nutrition for healthy sperm

A well-balanced diet is essential for sperm health, and certain key nutrients boost sperm production and neutralize damage. Your partner should take a good multivitamin and mineral supplement to maintain supplies of these vital nutrients, and he should also think about how to include them in his diet.

Amino acids

These are the building blocks of proteins and are essential if sperm are to mature properly. They are found in protein foods (see page 55), but I recommend that your partner also takes a supplement.

An important amino acid is L-arginine. In one study, sperm counts doubled after supplements were taken. The head of the sperm contains a large amount of L-arginine and this amino acid is essential for sperm production.

Overall, clinical trials confirm its effectiveness at levels of 500mg a day, although the benefits may be less in men with extremely low counts. Do not take arginine supplements if you have the herpes virus – it can stimulate an attack.

Other important amino acids include L-carnitine, essential for the normal functioning of sperm (50mg a day recommended); and taurine, which is found in high levels in sperm and is needed for good motility (50mg).

Vitamin A

This vitamin is essential for the production of male sex hormones. Animal research shows that deficiency may produce degeneration of the seminiferous tubules (see page 14), reduced semen volume and sperm count, and abnormal sperm morphology. For good food sources, see page 59.

Take vitamin A supplements with foods containing fat or oil. Adequate protein foods, as well as vitamins C and E and zinc, and proper thyroid function, are needed to mobilize vitamin A from the liver for transportation around the body.

▶ **Dosage** RNI men 700mcg/day.

Vitamin B6

Together with zinc, vitamin B6 is essential for the formation of male sex hormones. Deficiency has been found to cause infertility in studies of animals. See page 60 for food sources of vitamin B6 and pages 59–60 for information about how to supplement B vitamins.

▶ **Dosage** RNI men 1.4mg/day, but I would recommend 50mg a day.

Vitamin B12

Vitamin B12 is needed, together with folate (folic acid), for the synthesis of DNA and RNA. These are important compounds that are part of our genetic blueprint and are involved in the make-up of every cell in the body. B12 also helps with the uptake of folate.

Low levels of B12 are associated with abnormal sperm production, reduced sperm counts and reduced sperm motility. Even if there is no deficiency, supplementation is worthwhile in men with sperm counts of less than 20 million/ml. In one study, 27 per cent of men who had sperm counts of less than 20 million and were given B12 injections every day achieved counts in excess of 100 million/ml.

The only reliable sources of B12 are animal products, in particular lamb, sardines and salmon. Vegans should eat fermented foods that contain bacteria, but it is better to take supplements to ensure adequate intakes. Calcium aids the absorption of vitamin B12. See pages 59–60 for information about how to supplement B vitamins.

▶ **Dosage** RNI men 1.5mcg/day.

Folate (folic acid)

Folate is very important for all rapidly dividing cells, and for the production of healthy sperm. It improves sperm count and sperm motility as well as reducing the number of morphological abnormalities. Research has shown that folic acid is just as important a nutrient for men as it is for women, and folate deficiency may be a contributing factor to male infertility in as many as 10 per cent of cases. See page 61 for good

Healthy sperm emerging from a network of tiny tubes linked to the seminiferous tubules (see page 14) where sperm are produced.

food sources and information about taking folic acid supplements.

▶ **Dosage** RNI men 200mcg/day, but I would recommend taking 400mcg/day.

Vitamin C

Vitamin C is needed for the development of healthy sperm. Research in 1991 found that men with low levels of vitamin C were more likely to have genetically damaged sperm. This may not affect fertility directly, but any genetic damage to sperm would increase the risk of a child being born with a birth defect. Vitamin C is an antioxidant. It blocks the action of free-oxidizing radicals, which can cause gene damage.

Many studies have found that vitamin C supplementation can improve sperm motility. 200mg/day taken for four weeks increases sperm count as well as motility. Vitamin C also prevents the sperm from clumping together.

See page 61 for food sources of Vitamin C.

▶ **Dosage** RNI men 40mg/day, but I would recommend 1000mg/day.

Vitamin E

This vitamin is important for fertility. In 1922 researchers found that male rats fed on a vitamin E-free diet were unable to reproduce, but fertility returned when wheat-germ oil was added to their diet. As a major antioxidant, vitamin E helps to protect the high level of polyunsaturated fatty acids found in sperm cell membranes from damage by free-oxidizing radicals. In one study, 400IU of vitamin E given to men twice daily for three months led to a significant improvement in their sperm's ability to bind to and penetrate an egg. Severe vitamin E deficiency can lead to degeneration of the testicular tissue. If this damage becomes permanent, vitamin E

Leafy vegetables provide many nutrients, such as folate, calcium, magnesium, potassium, iron, PABA and vitamins A, B2, B6 and E.

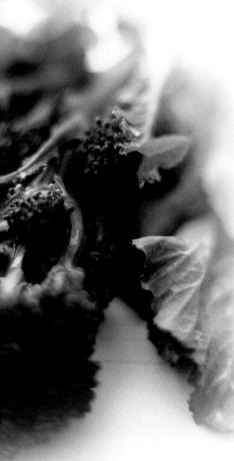

supplements are not able to repair it and a man will become sterile.

A natural (d-alpha-tocopherol), as opposed to synthetic (dl-alpha-tocopherol), supplement of this vitamin is more easily utilized by the body and retained for longer in the body tissues. Check the packet when buying a supplement to see which it is. See page 61 for main food sources and information about supplementing vitamin E.

▶ **Dosage** RNI men >4mg.

Selenium

Selenium is needed to form normally shaped sperm and to maintain a normal sperm count. Low levels of this mineral in semen have been linked to infertility. Studies on rats indicate that selenium is vitally important for the proper functioning of the epididymis (see pages 14–15), which is related to sperm maturation and motility.

Selenium also has antioxidant properties, protecting cells with a high lipid (fat) content in semen against possible damage from free radicals. See page 63 for food sources and information about how to supplement selenium.

▶ **Dosage** RNI men 75mcg/day.

Manganese

Manganese deficiency in animals can lead to testicular degeneration and congenital malformations. Tests on animals have found that males with severe manganese deficiency exhibit sterility and an absence of libido, low sperm

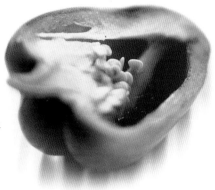

Red peppers are full of the essential vitamins A, C and E.

count and increasing numbers of degenerating cells in the epididymis. A lack of manganese may inhibit the synthesis of sex hormones, and possibly other steroids (important organic compounds in the body), with consequent infertility. See page 63 for food sources and information about supplementing manganese.

▶ **Dosage** RNI men 1.4mg/day.

Zinc

One of the nutrients most commonly lacking in the modern-day diet, zinc is vital for the production of healthy sperm. It is the most critical trace mineral involved in male sexual function, and is used in virtually every aspect of reproduction, including testosterone metabolism, testicle growth and sperm production. It is also important for the motility of sperm and a good sperm count. Zinc also helps reduce excessive amounts of oestrogen in male reproductive tissue, a factor that is linked to low sperm count.

Zinc is about 30 times more concentrated in sperm than in the bloodstream, and is largely found in the sperm head. Every time a man ejaculates, he loses about 5mg of this vitally important mineral.

A lot of research has shown that supplementing zinc improves fertility, and many studies suggest that 30mg a day will guard against deficiency, help to normalize sperm count, improve sperm motility and increase testosterone production. See page 63 for good food sources and information about how to supplement zinc.

▶ **Dosage** RNI men 9.5mg/day.

Co-enzyme Q10

Co-enzyme Q10, a fat-soluble vitamin-like substance found in every cell of the body, is present in large amounts in seminal fluid. It helps to protect sperm from damage by free radicals and supercharges them with energy, increasing their motility.

It is difficult to obtain sufficient amounts of co-enzyme Q10 from food sources (although it has been found that vegetarians have higher levels in their bodies than meat-eaters), so supplementation is the only reliable way of boosting your intake. There are no recommended intake levels for co-enzyme Q10, but I usually suggest between 50mg and 90mg a day.

Essential fatty acids

Essential fatty acids act as hormone regulators and the body cannot function without them. I believe it is vitally important to take them as a supplement.

Prostaglandins are made up of EFAs, and these are important for hormone regulation. Sperm contain high concentrations of omega-3 EFAs, particularly DHA (decosahexaenoic acid), the fatty acid found in oily fish. Most DHA is in the sperm tail and is thought to be important for sperm motility. Many men are deficient in omega-3 EFAs. Eating mackerel, herring, salmon or sardines at least two or three times a week (avoid tuna because of its high mercury levels), along with a daily supplement of 2000mg of EFA will help to improve this situation. Vegan-sourced DHA and EPA are available.

Very high levels of omega-6-derived prostaglandins are found in sperm cell membranes, and low levels of omega-6 EFAs are significantly linked to reduced male fertility. See page 64 for more details of food sources and information about how to supplement omega-3 and -6 EFAs.

EFAs are very prone to free-radical damage and good levels of antioxidants in the body are required to reduce this risk. See pages 59–63 for antioxidant nutrients – vitamins A, C and E and selenium.

PABA

Based on studies done as long ago as the 1940s, para-aminobenzoic acid (PABA) has been associated with male fertility – in support of the functioning of the pituitary gland and hence reproductive

hormones. A B-complex component, PABA may also be of benefit for folate production by intestinal bacteria, the production of red blood cells and the processing of proteins. Food sources of PABA include organ meats, whole grains, brewer's yeast, molasses, spinach and mushrooms. Folic acid and B-complex vitamins aid absorption; stress and antibiotics hinder it.

Herbs for men

Ginseng may improve levels of testosterone. Tribullus has been found to support healthy sperm production and is used to treat sexual dysfunction (impotence and lack of libido). Limited research has been done on certain herbs that are believed to have a negative effect on fertility. These include St John's wort, saw palmetto, liquorice and echinacea (see also page 36).

Walnuts are a valuable source of manganese and vitamin E, and release energy slowly for efficient use.

Countdown to conception

Now that you have improved your fertility status and become familiar with your menstrual cycle, you can give conception your best shot. The following pages will guide you through each phase of your cycle to maximize your chances of conceiving.

Massage will help you to relax
and avoid becoming overly anxious during the next month or so as you try to conceive and then wait to see if you are pregnant.

The conception plan

If, for the last few months, you and your partner have adopted the changes I have recommended to boost your fertility, you have given yourselves the best chance of conceiving. Now that you are trying to conceive, there are certain adjustments you can make each week during your cycle while keeping to the basics of healthy eating and living.

I work with clients to help them understand what is going on inside their bodies while they try to get pregnant. Over the next few pages I explain these changes and provide week-by-week guidelines on diet, lifestyle changes and complementary therapies to suit your body during each phase of the cycle.

Adjusting the plan

The average cycle is 28 days long, so the conception plan is divided into four weeks. Every woman is different, however, and many do not conform to this. Use the chart opposite to help you adjust the plan if your cycle is longer or shorter than 28 days.

Changing emotions

Once you and your partner decide to start a family, everything is wonderful. Sex is fantastic because caution (and precautions) are thrown to the wind. But after a few months without conceiving, you might start to think you have a problem. A cycle of highs and lows begins – optimism around ovulation followed by disappointment when your period arrives. Then there is the worry that stress is sabotaging your chances of conceiving.

Adjusting the plan for longer or shorter cycles

The plan (see pages 80–91) is based on a 28-day cycle. If your cycle is longer or shorter, use this chart to work out how long to use the information for each week, and when you are ovulating.

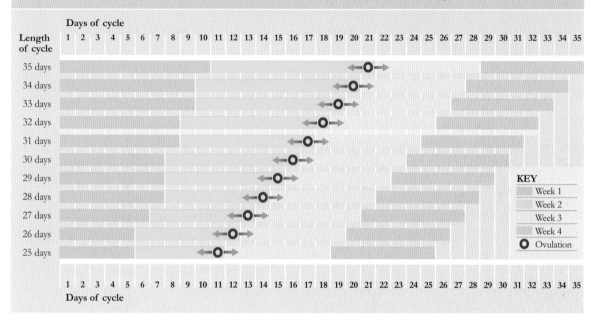

Days of cycle

Length of cycle	1	2	3	4	5	6	7	8	9	10	11	12	13	14	15	16	17	18	19	20	21	22	23	24	25	26	27	28	29	30	31	32	33	34	35

KEY

- Week 1
- Week 2
- Week 3
- Week 4
- O Ovulation

Avoiding anxiety

If you find yourself becoming anxious, try to relax. Remember the following points.

* Don't panic. Nature has its cycles (of dormancy in winter followed by new growth in spring). Although you can try to lend a helping hand, nature generally refuses to be rushed. Go with the flow a little.

* Don't assume you have a problem or dwell on the negative. Limit the amount of time you spend thinking about babies and pregnancy, and don't allow yourself to think about what isn't happening. Visualize a positive outcome and distract yourself from negative thoughts.

* Before you race to a fertility specialist, take a long hard look at yourselves and think "have we done everything possible to conceive naturally?" If you feel you have the time, give yourselves a few more months off trying while you make any improvements that you can to your lifestyle.

* Be patient. The statistics on rates of conception tell us that the average couple takes about nine months to a year to conceive.

* Keep your balance and perspective – take control of the situation (by following the countdown to conception plan on pages 82–91) rather than letting it control you.

This is an exciting time: enjoy it as much as you can. Keeping positive and cheerful can only improve your chances of conceiving.

If you are older or suspect you might have a fertility problem, it might help to pencil into your diary a date for making an appointment for you and your partner to see your doctor to talk about fertility testing. Until that date arrives, relax and let nature take its course. Just making that plan, knowing your alternatives and feeling you are taking positive action (with nutrition and exercise) can make a huge difference to your anxiety levels and relieve the heavy weight on your mind.

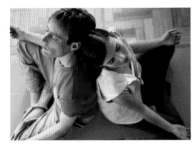

Week 1
at a glance

Chart your cycle

Oestrogen

Progesterone   KEY

| | Fertile phase |
| | Ovulation |

Menstruation

| 1 | 8 | 15 | 22 | 28 |

Cycle days 1–28

Focus on

DIET AND NUTRITION
Eat well – this is not the week to fast or diet. Avoid alcohol but drink plenty of water. Nutrients are needed (see opposite) to regenerate the endometrium, start the regrowth of follicles and balance hormones.

LIFESTYLE
In ancient cultures, menstruation was a time for women to withdraw from society and rest. You may not feel like being sociable at this time. The modern world doesn't stop for menstruating women, but in a hectic life, you should make space and time to reflect and be still.

The first week

Menstruation is the beginning of the follicular phase (see page 10), when follicles begin to grow. Chinese medicine regards the shedding of the lining of the uterus as the body cleansing itself: this is the inward and reflective *yin* phase of your cycle.

Menstruation

Hormones
Falling oestrogen and progesterone levels signal to the hypothalamus to release GnRH (gonadotrophin-releasing hormone), which triggers bleeding. This, in turn, prompts the pituitary to release FSH (follicle-stimulating hormone), which will start the growth of follicles and the development of an egg inside each of them.

The majority of women begin a period at night or within the first four hours of waking. How long bleeding lasts varies from woman to woman, but it is generally between five and seven days, with the heaviest bleeding on the first day. The outer two-thirds of the lining is shed gradually. The endometrium starts to regenerate within two days of the start of menstruation and by day five is already 2mm (1/16in) thick.

According to Traditional Chinese Medicine, bleeding should last for 3–5 days. Flow should be not too heavy, nor too light – around 50–80ml (2–3fl oz) is optimum, although the exact quantity is hard to gauge, and what some women

consider to be heavy bleeding is quite normal for others.

In the West, period pain is regarded as normal, and many women take painkillers routinely. In Chinese medicine, it is regarded as an indication of an obstruction in the flow of blood and *qi* (see page 72), both of which should be smooth. Blood should be bright red in colour: dark or brown blood is old blood. Pink blood is thin and poor quality, while clots indicate stagnation in the flow.

Lifestyle
The body's energy naturally ebbs during a period. Don't fight this tiredness: allow yourself to rest. Soak in a warm, candlelit bath and have a few early nights, allowing your vital energy to be used for the regeneration to come.

It is good to be inward-looking rather than outgoing at this time. Use the time for reflection and visualization. Think positively about moving on to a new cycle and a new attempt to conceive. Accept the fact that for now, at least, you are not pregnant, and look at what improvements you can make for the month ahead. Make sure you keep the lower abdomen, which the Chinese call the lower chou, warm at all times.

Chinese medicine does not recommend sex during a woman's period since it affects the blood flow. Research shows that many women, in fact, don't want sex during their period.

Diet and nutrition

Continue all the good nutritional habits you have established during the last few months. Make sure that you are getting all the vitamins, minerals and trace elements you need for this part of your cycle.

* Vitamins A and E, selenium and bioflavonoids are all important for building up the endometrium. See pages 59–64 for dosage and good food sources.
* Eating foods rich in iron (with vitamin C to aid absorption) will help to compensate for blood loss. See pages 59–63 for dosages and good food sources.
* Take a supplement of co-enzyme Q10 (see pages 59–63) to help oxygenate the blood and improve blood circulation generally.
* Vitamin B1 is important for building up the blood. See page 60 for dosages and food sources.

Exercise

Avoid strenuous or aerobic exercise during your period. Consider doing yoga, meditation or qi gong, an ancient system of movement, breathing and meditation. Dao yin breathing (see page 44) may also be of benefit. Don't go swimming at this time because, according to traditional Chinese beliefs, the abdomen will get cold.

Complementary therapies

Acupuncture can help to regulate the blood flow, build up your *qi* and relieve pain. Different points will be used depending on whether blood flow needs to be increased (if it is too light) or reduced (if too heavy).

Moxabustion (the burning of small cones of dried mugwort or moxa to warm up certain acupoints) may also be used to build up the blood. In Chinese medicine, the important organs for reproduction are the kidneys, heart and uterus. The nature and quality of blood flow is a vital diagnostic tool, and your acupuncturist will ask you about the amount, colour, consistency and degree of clotting. Pain is also significant – lower back pain, for example, is a sign of kidney deficiency. Make notes of all your menstrual details to take along.

Acupressure can also help blood flow and may be self-administered. Press gently but firmly for five minutes twice a day on the acupoints Large Intestine 4 (in the triangle formed by the thumb and index finger) and Spleen 6 (three finger breadths above the ankle bone on the inside leg).

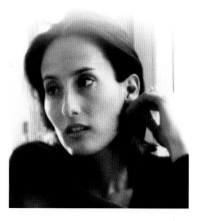

Your emotions

For many women, this is a difficult week because their period brings confirmation that they are not pregnant. **It can be a low point, filled with despair, anger, frustration and hopelessness.** As negative as you may feel, remember that your body is cleansing itself before regenerating.

Many cultures view the period as physical renewal – the body prepares for a fresh cycle. Cleanse yourself mentally and emotionally, too. Don't feel guilty about the odd glass of wine you may have had.

You're low in energy and feel introverted, but feel a lightening from your premenstrual mood.

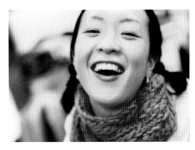

Week 2
at a glance

Chart your cycle

Oestrogen

Progesterone

Menstruation

KEY
Fertile phase
Ovulation

1   8   15   22   28

Cycle days 1–28

Focus on

DIET
Diet is crucially important to hormonal balance and good egg quality. Once ovulation, fertilization and implantation occur, everything happens quickly. You need certain nutrients to ensure that the uterus is prepared and cell division is successful. If you have deficiencies, take supplements (see opposite).

LIFESTYLE
You will feel more energetic this week than last week and you will be much more inclined to do exercise. It's fine to keep to your normal exercise routine (see also page 86).

The second week

This is the most important time of the month from the point of view of fertility. Between 10 and 20 egg follicles have been developing, but only one of them will become dominant this week. The rest will gradually degenerate. By the time of ovulation, which takes place at the end of this week, only the one dominant follicle will remain.

Ovulation

Hormones
Follicle-stimulating hormone (FSH) levels rise to stimulate further the growth and ripening of the follicles. Initially these are about 4mm (⅛in) in diameter, but by the time of ovulation they will be five times bigger. By day nine, there will be twice as many blood vessels in a dominant follicle as in the other follicles. The rising FSH levels prompt the ovaries to release oestrogen, which starts the renewal and thickening of the endometrium (ready for possible implantation).

As oestrogen levels rise, FSH levels fall so that no more eggs mature. Oestrogen levels peak at around day 12, sending a signal to the hypothalamus to release luteinizing hormone (LH).

LH triggers changes in the ovary and follicle that will lead up to ovulation. With the LH surge around day 14, one part of the outer membrane of the follicle starts to thin. Within another 24–36 hours, the follicle membrane ruptures and the egg and its surrounding follicular fluid are released.

After ovulation the egg is swept into the Fallopian tube to begin its journey towards the uterus. Fertilization occurs in the middle section of the tube.

Diet and nutrition

Ensure that your body has all the nourishment it needs during this vitally important week of the cycle. Continue to follow the healthy eating programme as you have been for the last few months but pay particular attention to certain essential nutrients.

* All the B vitamins are important for the release of the egg, then, if it is fertilized, its implantation in the lining of the uterus and the early development of an embryo. See pages 59–61 for dosages and good food sources of all B vitamins. Vitamin B12 in particular (see page 60) is needed for the synthesis of DNA and RNA, the materials that make up the genetic blueprint of a human being and which are present in the nucleus of every egg.

* Zinc, magnesium, selenium and vitamin A are all essential nutrients for egg production, and zinc is also needed to promote cell division. Eat plenty of foods rich in these nutrients during this week. See pages 59–63 for dosages and good food sources of these essential nutrients.

* Vitamin C helps to replenish the ovaries and, together with vitamin E, selenium and zinc, is present in the follicular fluid surrounding an egg. These essential nutrients are believed to nourish the egg during its development. See pages 61–63 for good food sources and recommended daily intakes.

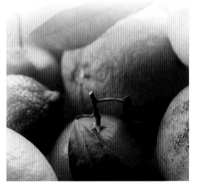

Vitamin C is an antioxidant that helps to "mop up" potentially harmful debris in the reproductive system.

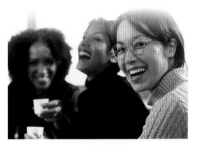

Your emotions

Studies show that increased levels of oestrogen increase your sense of wellbeing. Clients tell me they feel full of anticipation now as they can "try again". You feel slimmer and more attractive. **Your energy levels rise and you feel more dynamic and outgoing** than last week. You are focused on goals and full of enthusiasm, positivity and new ideas. It is a time of mental and physical activity, when ideas you may have had last week start to take on structure. Sexual desire peaks as ovulation approaches, and you feel "creative" at every level. As much as you reach a high at this point, try to focus on your secretions and what is happening to your body.

Key indicators of ovulation

Look out for the following signs and symptoms, as they may indicate that ovulation has occurred. Don't worry if you fail to pick up any of these signs: it doesn't mean you haven't ovulated.

* Abundant cervical secretions are a sign that you are at your most fertile – the secretions will be watery, stretchy and transparent (see pages 70–71).

* Your desire for sexual intercourse will increase markedly this week.
* A slight rise in body temperature after ovulation will last from now until your next bleed (if there is one).
* Ovulation pain (or Mittelschmerz as it is called) is something many women experience – it is a dull ache on one side of the lower abdomen, and lasts anything from a few minutes to several hours.

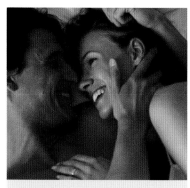

When to have sex

There are many myths surrounding sex and a lot of confusion and misinformation about the best time to have sex in order to conceive. I am amazed to discover that many of my clients either do not have enough sex or do it at the wrong time.

Sperm can usually survive for quite a long time – up to 3–5 days in alkaline secretions (and even as long as seven days), waiting for the egg to arrive. An egg is fertilizable for up to 24 hours. So the best time to have sex is during the time leading up to ovulation, when your secretions are at their most fertile: wetter, clearer, more transparent and stretchy.

Some women become very anxious, thinking that the egg only lasts a number of hours, because their own work commitments or their partner's plans are not compatible with their time of ovulation. This can be very stressful for the woman desperate to conceive and a big turn-off for the man expected to "perform" no matter what.

Exercise

Make the most of feeling fully alive by taking some brisk walks and regular aerobic exercise to get your *qi* circulating. Go running, swimming, power walking, cycling or visit the gym.

Complementary therapies

Use the aromatherapy oils sandalwood, jasmine or ylang-ylang, which are believed to have aphrodisiac qualities. Only use these in oil burners or in scented candles, however – do not put them on your skin either by adding oil to your bath water or using one as a massage oil, since this will interfere with your body's own pheromones. Male and female bodies give off

At fertilization, a sperm penetrates the egg, dissolving its outer coating in a chemical reaction.

natural odours that, some people believe, shouldn't be interfered with. You may not want to use perfume or other scented products for the same reason.

I recommend acupuncture as close to ovulation as possible. The acupoint is the Door of Infants on the lower abdomen (see diagram on page 73). An acupuncturist will tell you your individual pattern of disharmony and use points suitable to you.

Visualization

Make time this week to visualize the processes of ovulation and fertilization. Picture the egg being released as the follicle ruptures (see picture on page 170). The egg then oozes out onto the surface of the ovary. It is now sitting on the surface, surrounded by a mass of sticky cells known as the cumulus oophorous. These cells play a crucial role, making it possible for the Fallopian tube to pick up the egg. The egg is gathered up by fimbria, which are finger-like projections at the end of each Fallopian tube, and swept into the tube. From here it moves towards the uterus during the next seven days, helped by cilia, tiny hairs lining the Fallopian tubes. Fertilization takes place when a successful sperm, which has swum up through the cervix and uterus and into the Fallopian tube, penetrates the egg. This happens in what is known as the distal third of the tube – that is, the section closest to the ovary. The fertilized egg, now known as a zygote (see page 13), continues its journey towards the uterus.

Sex under pressure

Sexual problems can often develop at this time. Men feel that the sexual act has become a very mechanical means to an end. Women become obsessive about having sex at just the right time so that the sperm can "get ahead" and be in place waiting for the egg. Tensions are running high, and I have often heard from my clients how all this stress can lead to arguments and hence no sex. Try not to put yourselves under such pressure and enjoy what you are doing for its own sake.

Zita's tips

* **You cannot have too much sex.** Contrary to what many people believe, frequent sex does not somehow weaken the sperm. In fact, fertility is improved by frequent intercourse. Research has shown that couples having sex once a week have a 15 per cent chance of conceiving during a cycle, whereas those making love every day increased that chance to 50 per cent. So, aim to have lots of passionate sex at least two or three times a week.

* **Remember: you are designed** to have maximum sexual desire when you are at your most fertile. You will be able to detect this from your secretions (see pages 70–71). Many women try to pinpoint ovulation accurately. This is neither possible (without a scan) nor necessary. Ovulation predictor kits identify the LH (luteinizing hormone) surge about 24 hours before ovulation and temperature charts will show a temperature rise after ovulation.

* **Touch and caress each other** prior to intercourse, as sexual stimulation increases the flow of hormones and encourages fertility. Studies show that the sperm count of ejaculate from men who were turned on by a partner is higher and more potent than that of ejaculate from men who masturbated.

* **Don't use artificial lubricants in the vagina, unless sperm-friendly.** Oils, water-based gels and even saliva can adversely affect the motility of sperm. The best lubrication is your own arousal fluids, which will be plentiful if you have lots of sexual stimulation prior to having intercourse.

* **Aim for sexual positions** that involve deep penetration if you want to encourage the greatest amount of contact between sperm and secretions.

* **Stay in bed for 20 minutes after intercourse** to encourage the sperm to stay in your vagina. Strong swimmers will quickly find their way through the fertile cervical secretions and move up into the uterus towards the Fallopian tubes. Weaker sperm will inevitably stay in the vagina, and there will eventually be flow back from your body whatever position you adopt. There is no need to stand on your head!

* **Avoid going to the loo** for 20–30 minutes after intercourse.

* **Do not use recreational drugs or alcohol.** There is mounting evidence to show that the presence of drugs or alcohol in the blood of either partner can have a negative impact on fertility generally and conception.

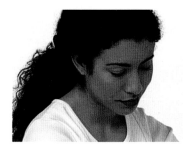

Week 3
at a glance

Chart your cycle

Oestrogen

Progesterone

KEY
Fertile phase
Ovulation

Menstruation

| 1 | 8 | 15 | 22 | 28 |

Cycle days 1–28

Focus on

DIET
Make sure that you maintain your good dietary habits but consider boosting certain nutrients (see right), either by supplementation or in your food. If fertilization has occurred, you may be about to be eating for two.

LIFESTYLE
Keep the *qi* flowing smoothly in your body (see page 72). Take at least 20 minutes of moderate exercise at least three times a week. Spend time each day calmly and positively visualizing the implantation process in your uterus (see page 43 and opposite).

The third week

This week marks the start of the waiting time, as you wonder what is going on inside your body and hope that fertilization takes place and that implantation will occur successfully.

Fertilization

Your hormones
Last week, as soon as ovulation took place, levels of FSH (follicle-stimulating hormone) began to drop sharply and LH (luteinizing hormone) levels began to fall slowly. Now it is the time for progesterone to play an important role. This next phase of the cycle is the luteal phase (see pages 10–11). It needs to last for a minimum of nine days. If less, there will be insufficient time for implantation to take place so that, even if fertilization has occurred, the pregnancy may fail.

The follicle that contained the egg, having ruptured, remained behind. It still received pulses of LH, which continue this week. This enables it to turn into a small cyst or corpus luteum (literally "yellow body", see pages 10–11), which produces progesterone.

Progesterone has four important functions to perform at this stage of the cycle:
* it helps to build and thicken the lining of the uterus so that it can secrete nutrients that will provide the developing embryo with nourishment

* it switches off the production of FSH and LH to prevent more eggs from ripening
* it raises basal body temperature by 0.2°C (32.4°F) in order to help prepare the uterus for receiving the embryo
* it closes the cervix and thickens the mucus, forming a plug to prevent more sperm entering the cervix after fertilization.

Diet and nutrition
In order for the egg to travel down the Fallopian tube and divide, a good supply of nutrients is needed.
* Zinc is very important for cell division and the production of progesterone. See page 63 for dosage and good food sources of zinc.
* Vitamin A is also important for progesterone production and to protect a developing embryo. See page 59 for dosage and good food sources of vitamin A.
* Vitamin C is highly concentrated in the corpus luteum so it is believed to be linked to the

release of progesterone. See page 61 for dosage and good food sources of vitamin C.

Lifestyle changes

Many of you reading this may have been trying to conceive for months and feel as if you have put your life on hold. This might be invoking a sense of urgency in you, which may make you behave a bit obsessively. Try to practise moderation in all things and don't become obsessive about what you can and can't allow yourself to do.

Exercise

Traditional Chinese Medicine works on the premise that it is important to get the *qi* circulating at this stage so as to get the egg moving into the uterus. Take moderate exercise such as walking or cycling, but avoid excessive aerobic exercise.

Complementary therapies

Acupuncture can be very effective throughout your cycle when you are trying to conceive, but especially in the 6–8 days after ovulation. I treat clients to remove imbalances and promote the healthy flow of *qi*. Two points needled at this time are Gate of Life and Door of Infants (see page 73). Your acupuncturist might use moxabustion to warm the lower chou (lower abdomen).

Visualization

Concentrate on the details of what is hopefully happening inside you. The developing embryo continues its journey along the Fallopian tube towards the uterus. The corpus luteum continues to secrete progesterone and maintain a fairly constant level of oestrogen. Progesterone levels continue to rise and influence the lining of the uterus. This thickens, in readiness for receiving the embryo and supporting it once it has embedded. By about day 21 (of a 28-day cycle), the embryo – by now a multi-celled blastocyst (see illustration below) – embeds into the wall of the uterus, burrowing into the nourishing cells and eventually connecting with the maternal blood supply. You may experience slight spotting a week or so after ovulation.

A six- or seven-day-old blastocyst embeds itself into the plump, nutrient-rich lining of the uterus.

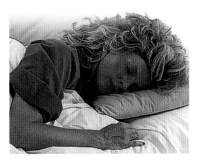

Your emotions

Hope and anticipation are familiar emotions this week, as is anxiety, as you wonder whether or not all has gone well and you could be pregnant.

Since last week, hormones have had a positive influence on your mood, making you feel energetic and positive. But if you are trying to conceive, all this good feeling may be overshadowed by the pressure of waiting until you can take a pregnancy test. Once ovulation has passed, the outgoing feelings tend to turn inward and you become reflective and emotional. Women tend to dream more vividly at this stage of the month, as if their unconscious is demanding to be listened to.

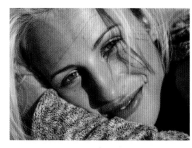

The fourth week

As the waiting game creeps towards the pregnancy test, the pressure continues to mount this week. Work on keeping yourself calm and serene. It's important to hope for the best and stay positive.

Week 4
at a glance

Chart your cycle

Oestrogen

Progesterone

KEY
Fertile phase
Ovulation

Menstruation

| 1 | 8 | 15 | 22 | 28 |

Cycle days 1–28

Focus on

DIET AND NUTRITION

As during the preceding weeks, you should maintain the healthy eating patterns you established during your programme of preconceptual care because, if you are pregnant, you now need those nutrients (see pages 59–64) to nourish a baby.

LIFESTYLE

Exercise will help you focus on something other than whether or not you might be pregnant, and more holistic and reflective forms of activity might prevent you from tearing your hair out by relaxing your body and calming your mind.

Development or degeneration

Hormones

An embryo arrives in the uterus approximately 4–5 days after fertilization, and implantation occurs about 7–10 days after ovulation (in a 28-day cycle). The more developed the blastocyst before it implants, the greater the chance of a successful pregnancy. An embryo has about 30 cells by the time it reaches the uterus, and it starts to break out of its surrounding membrane, the zona pellucida. As women age, the zona becomes tougher and it is therefore more difficult for the embryo to hatch out. (IVF fertility treatment may include assisted hatching, whereby the "shell" is broken slightly to allow the embryo to emerge.)

Once implantation has occurred, the developing placental tissues start to produce the pregnancy hormone HCG (human chorionic gonadotrophin). This maintains the structure of the endometrium and the continued existence of the corpus luteum (see pages 10–12), which produces increasing quantities of progesterone in order to sustain the pregnancy for the next 12 weeks until the placenta has fully developed and is ready to take over pregnancy maintenance.

If conception hasn't taken place, the corpus luteum will survive for 12–16 days after ovulation, then it will degenerate. The endometrium, which is about 8–10mm (⅜–½in) thick by now, stops developing any further and the uterus prepares to shed the lining. Falling levels of oestrogen and progesterone trigger the hypothalamus to release GnRH (gonadotrophin-releasing hormone) and FSH (follicle-stimulating hormone), which begin the cycle of bleeding and the development of follicles again.

Diet and nutrition

Within your established dietary programme (see box, left), you should pay particular attention to include foods containing essential fatty acids (EFAs), vitamins B6 and E, zinc and magnesium. For good food sources, see pages 60–64.

The Chinese believe that at this time you should eat plenty of warming *yang* foods. These should include as little raw food as possible and up to two litres (3.5 pints) of water (at room temperature) a day. Any fresh juices should be made from fruits and vegetables kept at room temperature. If you eat a salad, have something warming with it, such as a jacket potato, or eat the salad as an accompaniment to a hot dish. Foods should be warming and easy to digest, such as soups, casseroles, well-cooked meats, lentils, porridge, potatoes and sweet potatoes, papaya, ginger and barley. Other *yang* foods include chicken, eggs, mushrooms, sesame oil, peanuts, garlic and onions and red foods such as tomatoes and sweet peppers. If, as the week wears on, you begin to suspect that you might be about to start a period, follow dietary guidelines to maximize hormonal balance (see page 126).

Exercise

By all means carry on as normal with exercise this week, but, if you think you might be pregnant, don't engage in high-impact, aerobic activities that involve any bouncing. Pilates, brisk walking, yoga, cycling or swimming are fine.

Complementary therapies

Deep breathing techniques (see pages 42–43) and visualization (see page 43) will encourage the embedded embryo to develop in the best possible way. The Chinese believe that wherever your mind is, *qi* will follow. Place your hand on your lower abdomen to see if it feels cold; if so, use a covered hot-water bottle to warm it up. Warmth is essential if you are to "grow" a baby.

Focus your energy on promoting inner calm as you approach the potential stress of a pregnancy test.

Your emotions

This can be an anxious time as you wait to see if your period will arrive and try to interpret your body's signals. Many women report feeling emotional and tearful at this time. **Try to focus your energies outwards rather than turning in on yourself.** You need to think positively, of course – that you might be pregnant. As the week progresses, however, you may start to experience what might be your familiar premenstrual symptoms recurring or, on the other hand, what might be the first signs of pregnancy. **You will need to reconcile these conflicting thoughts and then, if your period does come, you will be able to look forward (see pages 82–83). Don't forget to treat** yourself kindly – have a glass of wine if you feel like it – and spoil yourself a bit.

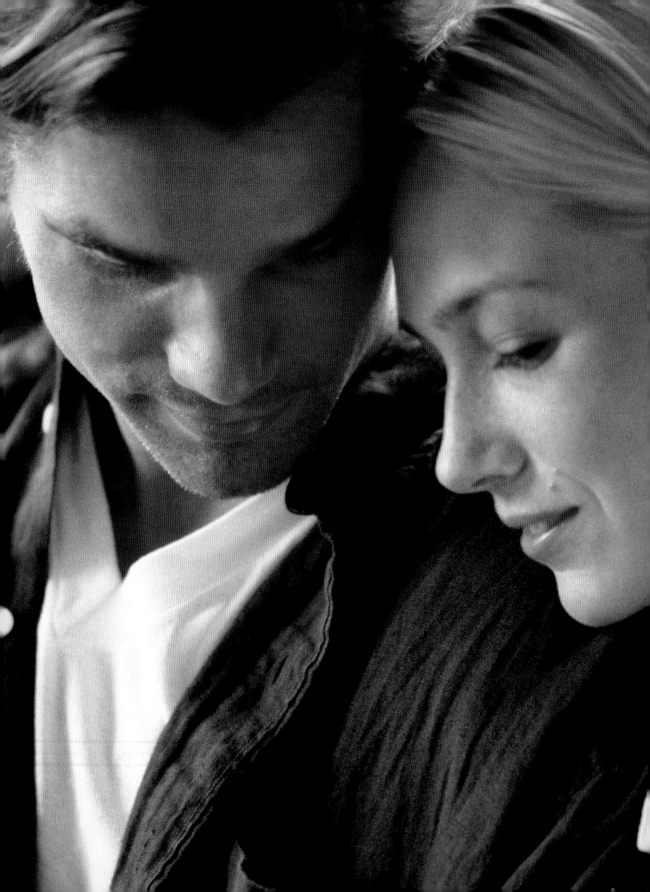

Testing your fertility

Over the past few months, you may have made many *lifestyle changes* to enhance your fertility and been making a *concerted effort to conceive* a baby, but so far *without success.* If you feel that you have done everything to maximize your chances of conceiving and suspect that you may have a *fertility problem,* you have reached the point at which you and your partner should make an appointment with your doctor to *discuss fertility tests. It's time for plan B.*

Moving forwards

If, after months of trying to conceive, you feel there is a problem, you will want to find out what it is and what can be done about it. You and your partner need to research all the options and work out a plan of action. Take things one step at a time, keep talking to each other and prepare for what lies ahead.

Thinking about plan B

How long do you try unsuccessfully for a baby before approaching your doctor? If you are aged between 20 and 35, try for 12 months before testing; if you are over 35, try for six months.

When a couple suspects that they might have a problem that is preventing them from conceiving, they usually feel apprehensive, wondering what the problem might be and often fearing the worst. They don't know what to expect from the testing process, fearing the unknown. Feel reassured by the tests, however. Many fertility problems are minor and can be dealt with relatively easily. If you are worried, you can start testing – with blood tests and sperm analysis – while continuing to try for a baby. Generally speaking, a couple with unexplained infertility have a similar chance of conceiving a baby during a 12-month period whether or not they have fertility treatment.

Talking to friends, family or a counsellor may help to relieve some of the pressure you're under.

Wrestling with emotions

You may well be experiencing a confusing variety of thoughts and emotions (see box, right), which can increase your stress levels and take a huge toll on your physical wellbeing. At this stage, my clients commonly feel and express any of the following emotions:

* **shock** "I never expected to be in this situation"
* **denial** "this can't be happening to me"
* **fear** "what if I never become pregnant?"
* **regret** "perhaps I've waited too long"
* **grief** "I may be unable to have the one thing I feel is essential to my life"
* **responsibility** "I've let my partner down"
* **isolation** "I feel I don't fit in among my friends any more. I want to avoid social gatherings in order to escape thoughtless remarks and questions….and other people's babies"
* **frustration and anger** "other people don't seem to have any problems getting pregnant: why should it be me who has the problems?"
* **envy** "I feel jealous of other couples when I see them with their babies"
* **failure** "there's something wrong with me – it's as though I'm defective or disabled in some way"
* **helplessness** "I have no control over my body and my future has been taken away"
* **anxiety** "how will we be able to afford fertility treatment, and will I be able to take enough time off work for all the consultations and tests?"
* **apprehension** "how will I get on with the drugs if I have to have fertility treatment?"

Talking about your feelings

It is difficult for most people to appreciate what you are going through unless they themselves have been in the same situation. Explain to friends and family how you are feeling and ask them for their support and understanding. If you find it hard to tell them face to face, perhaps write them a short note or e-mail describing how difficult it is for you both at the moment. Remind them, if you like, that stress does not cause infertility but infertility does cause stress,

Susan's thoughts

*"I am frustrated! I have always been healthy, but **all the time I am not getting pregnant I worry in case I don't 'work' properly.** I just want to know whether or not I can conceive. If I can't, I want to know what to do about it; if I can, then I can keep trying without the added anxiety of wondering whether or not it's possible.*

***I think the most frustrating part of this whole process is that I have no clue when it will happen, why it will happen or not, or what I can really do to make it happen.** It all seems quite out of my control. It is difficult to manage this process as I have become quite obsessive about it. Pregnancy is constantly on my mind and I try not to think about it too much as I don't want to get too wound up about it but it is hard to control my mind. It is challenging because everyone says that it will only happen when I am relaxed about it, but it is difficult not to be stressed about it as we have been trying for over a year now. **I worry that my anxiety and stress is preventing me from getting pregnant.** I don't talk about it with too many people because they all throw lots of advice at me, and I find it hard to navigate my way through all the advice, rumours and myths."*

Other sources of support

* **Check out some of the fertility websites,** and even chatrooms, on the internet. See Useful Websites on page 187 for details.

* **Enquire at your doctor's surgery** to see if there are any fertility support groups in your area.

* **Talk to women who are going through,** or who have been through, the same experience. This will make you feel far less isolated, and they will give you some idea of what to expect from tests and treatments.

and that no amount of relaxation will unblock blocked tubes or remove feelings of desperation. If you have difficulty dealing with some of your feelings, consider going to talk to a counsellor. He or she might help you to be able to understand your emotions better.

Laying ghosts to rest

Also, you can explore whether or not there is anything in your psyche that might be preventing you from conceiving a baby. Such things as a previous termination, problems with or doubts about your relationship with your partner, a traumatic childhood experience or the pressure of being the main breadwinner may all have an impact at a deep level. If there are any issues that you feel need to be dealt with, now is the time to address them. A therapist or counsellor might be able to help you put your mind at rest.

A sense of perspective

Take strength and comfort from the fact that you and your partner are not the only ones finding it difficult to conceive. Couples rarely seem to share with other people the fact that they are having problems conceiving – it remains an intensely private experience. It may appear as if everyone around you is getting pregnant, and there are mothers with babies wherever you look, but in fact one in six couples has a problem conceiving.

Understanding your partner's emotions

Men can sometimes find it much harder than their female partners to get in touch with their feelings and then to share them. In addition, men and women often have very different attitudes to sharing private feelings with others. You and your partner may find you have reacted quite differently to your situation; while your first instinct might have been to confide in friends and family, your partner may not want to discuss the situation with anybody. It's important that you decide between you who you want to tell and how involved in the process you want family and friends to be.

The experience of not being able to have a baby exactly when you'd planned and dealing with the consequences of that, whatever the outcome, can strengthen the emotional bond between the two of you. Far from driving a wedge between you, it may bring you closer together. Many couples have admitted to me after their treatment that, with hindsight, they are grateful for this bonding experience that they would have missed had they been able to conceive straight away.

Nurturing your relationship

Despite your disappointment at the realization that conceiving a baby might be problematical, do remember that you and your partner are what matters in both the short and long term. Having a child in the future may not be a certainty for you and, if that is the case, a mutually supportive relationship is what will help you both to come to terms with that future. Find a balance between this and other features of your life, keep talking to each other and try also to keep a sense of perspective. As you embark on a programme of fertility treatment, it's all too easy to let it dominate every aspect of your life and thinking. Limit the amount of time you spend talking about the subject each day, and refrain from referring to it at all during the course of a day or evening you have set aside and planned for togetherness.

Remembering your sex life

Whatever you do, don't give up on sex. Many couples, once they have been locked into fertility treatment for some time, find that they have no sex life at all, and their relationship can suffer accordingly. By now, the idea of "making love" may well have flown out of the window, and sex becomes a mechanical act that happens only to an all-important schedule. The act no longer has anything to do with your feelings but is solely dictated by the timetable of your clinic. This lack of spontaneity can be a huge turn-off for men, who are expected to perform at the optimum moment no matter what.

Even after years of failure to conceive, it may still be possible in some instances to achieve a spontaneous pregnancy, so it makes sense to keep having regular sex – just in case.

Couples who choose to go down the IVF (in vitro fertilization) route and know that fertilization will take place in a laboratory may even start to feel that sex is redundant. Having IVF treatment does not mean, however, that you have to give up on intimacy, fun, passion and tenderness. Try to take time out occasionally – a weekend away perhaps – to breathe life back into your sexual relationship. Remember that infertility is only temporary and once it is behind you, you will still want a sexual relationship. So look after it!

Don't lose sight of the fact that, whether or not you have a baby, you share a loving relationship.

Starting the ball rolling

If you and your partner have come to the conclusion that you might have a fertility problem, the things that will be uppermost in your mind are the possible cause of the problem and what you can do about it. Start to draw up an action plan. Make sure you discuss everything with each other as you prepare for what might lie ahead.

If you are determined to get pregnant, then it's time to make an appointment with your doctor to discuss fertility testing. If you are in your late 30s or older, visit your doctor straight away or go directly to a fertility clinic. Don't be fobbed off: be assertive. You may be told to go away and try again for a few more months. Take your temperature chart along and describe everything that you have been doing. If you've followed all the advice in Plan A, insist that your doctor tests you now.

Taking control

Fertility tests take the form of a progressive series of checks to eliminate possible causes of infertility in both men and women. At each level of testing, the results will determine what the next stage of testing should be, so don't expect a clear path ahead. There is no reason why testing shouldn't start at the same time for both you and your partner. It is often the woman who starts the ball rolling when it comes to fertility testing, but I often advise the couples I see to begin with sperm analysis. It is relatively straightforward, non-invasive and may quickly eliminate one potential problem, thus saving you time.

Although tests follow a chronological order, every case is different. Your particular experience will depend on the nature of your fertility problems and which treatment is considered to be the most appropriate for you. The testing process begins with your doctor. Depending on your age and how long you have been trying to conceive, you may be referred to a fertility clinic. The procedures can be fraught because of the amount of time it takes to attend consultations and schedule tests, and then wait for the results. The process can take longer if you are using the National Health Service in the UK. Take it one step at a time; focus only on what you are doing at any particular time, and be prepared to move the goalposts if something is not working for you.

Understanding the testing process will make you feel more in control of what is happening and less alarmed by it. The following pages outline the tests you might have to undergo so that you are prepared for anything that you might come across.

Zita's tips

The following tips will help you and your partner feel in control of what is happening while you test your fertility – and perhaps receive treatment – and think positively.

* **Find out all your options** and then take things one step at a time.

* **Maintain a sense of perspective:** don't put your life on hold and think of nothing but pregnancy.

* **Look at the bigger picture:** you may feel you need to take a break for a while, but consider making an appointment with a clinic in advance and then, having made a decision, you can relax for a bit.

* **Remember that your relationship is important,** whatever happens. Stay close to one another and keep talking everything through.

* **Limit yourself** to one hour per day of dealing with fertility measures, and make time for your partner.

* **Don't pester each other** about what you should or shouldn't be doing. You may be one step ahead of your partner in charting the progress of your fertility planning and treatment in the coming months. Accept that fact now.

Female fertility tests

Fertility tests for women are more complicated and varied than they are for men because hormone levels fluctuate during the female cycle and their interaction is complex.

The aim of tests

Many different factors or combinations of factors may affect fertility. Tests aim to eliminate possible causes of problems. Most tests, even the invasive, surgical ones, are quite routine and shouldn't give you too much cause for concern. You need to be prepared, however, for the possibility that some results might be inconclusive.

A series of tests may be necessary before conclusions can be reached. The sequence is as follows:

* **level one** hormone assessment – to detect any ovulation problems
* **level two** tubal and uterine assessment – to check for physical barriers to conception
* **level three** immunological screening – to assess possible reactions of your immune system.

Level one: hormone assessment

Simple blood tests can detect hormone imbalance that may be affecting your fertility. One test done on days 2–4 of your cycle will give an indication of egg quality and your ovarian reserve (see pages 16 and 101). This is especially important for women over the age of 35. Other blood tests at this time measure oestradiol, LH, prolactin and thyroid hormone levels if necessary.

Another blood test on day 21 (of a 28-day cycle) will measure levels of progesterone and show if ovulation has occurred. The timing will vary if your cycle is longer or shorter than 28 days.

FSH

This is the hormone produced by the pituitary gland to stimulate the growth and development of ovarian follicles. The FSH (follicle-stimulating hormone) level on days 2–4 of your cycle is used as a baseline measurement of ovarian reserve and quality of eggs. Perimenopausal and menopausal women have elevated levels of FSH (see page 17). Levels of FSH may also fluctuate if you have irregular periods.

Oestradiol (E_2)

This is the main oestrogen hormone secreted by ovarian follicles, and is measured in a blood test on days 2–4 of your cycle. It is not routine unless it is anticipated that you will need fertility treatment. As follicles grow and mature they produce E_2, causing the endometrium to thicken. This hormone also helps balance FSH levels, preventing

A blood test is the first step in any investigation of female fertility problems.

In polycystic disease, ovarian follicles enlarge and fill with fluid. These cystic follicles will not release eggs.

them from getting too high. As a woman approaches menopause, she does not produce enough oestradiol so cannot balance FSH (follicle-stimulating hormone), which rises. Ideally, both FSH and E_2 levels should be low. High levels may indicate an ovarian cyst or a diminished ovarian reserve.

LH

Luteinizing hormone is released by the pituitary gland, stimulating ovulation (see page 10), the formation of the corpus luteum (see pages 10–11) and the synthesis of progesterone by the ovaries. A surge of LH midway through your cycle triggers ovulation. Luteinizing hormone is tested during days 2–4: high levels may indicate polycystic ovary syndrome (PCOS) – see pages 119–21.

Prolactin

This hormone is secreted by the pituitary gland. Its major purpose is to control milk production after childbirth, but it also stimulates the production of progesterone. Levels of this hormone also tend to be higher in the luteal phase of your cycle (see pages 10–11).

Prolactin is tested if PCOS is suspected. Levels that are higher than expected may interfere with ovulation or result in a reduced progesterone function, which will make it difficult for your body to maintain a pregnancy.

Thyroid hormones

Thyroid-stimulating hormone (TSH) is produced by the pituitary gland and is responsible for controlling thyroid function. This is important for all metabolic processes and hence the proper functioning of all body systems. TSH levels are often checked first in a fertility evaluation because an under-active thyroid is linked to infertility (see page 106). A TSH level that is beyond the expected range, combined with a level of thyroxine (T_4) that is below the expected range or even within it, is usually indicative of an under-active thyroid. If TSH levels are within the expected range but T_4 levels are below it, you are more likely to have a problem with the pituitary gland. (Low T_4 may indicate a diseased thyroid or a non-functioning pituitary gland that is not stimulating the thyroid to produce T_4.)

Androgens

Levels of male hormones are also assessed in the blood test at the beginning of your cycle to rule out the possibility of PCOS. This might suggest a state of hormonal imbalance in which the pituitary gland produces large amounts of luteinizing hormone (LH), preventing ovulation and causing the ovaries to secrete higher than expected levels of male hormones.

Progesterone

When a follicle releases its egg, it becomes a corpus luteum (see pages 10–11) and progesterone is produced. A blood test on day 21 of your cycle, measuring levels of progesterone, will indicate whether or not you are ovulating. This test should actually be carried out 7–10 days after ovulation has occurred, which is day 21 for women who have a regular, 28-day menstrual cycle, or seven days before your period if you do not have a 28-day cycle. If your cycle is unusual, discuss the calculation with your doctor. The test is slightly problematic since progesterone is secreted in pulses every 2–3 hours, so a single test may not give an accurate reading of the overall level and you may be required to retest. Some doctors believe the test is more accurate if it is done first thing in the morning.

This test is also used to identify a luteal phase defect (LPD – see page 30). This will reduce the role of progesterone in preparing the endometrium for implantation of a fertilized egg. If there is insufficient progesterone being secreted, the lining of the uterus will not be ready for implantation and a pregnancy will not be viable.

If your progesterone level is lower than the expected range, it may mean that you haven't ovulated in that cycle – you will need to be tested again.

Ovarian reserve tests

The AMH blood test measures levels of anti-mullerian hormone, as there is a correlation with AMH and your ovarian reserve. In combination with an ultrasound scan to check the number of antral follicles on both ovaries, this test will give an indication of potential fertility – the higher the number of antral follicles and blood level

of AMH, the better the fertility potential. However, this test cannot determine egg quality, nor can it be done if you have PCOS. Age is still the biggest factor when it comes to ovarian reserves declining (see pages 16–17).

Interpreting results

If blood tests indicate that you are not ovulating, your doctor will advise you of the most suitable treatment options. Hormonal imbalance can often be adjusted by medication or changes to nutrition and lifestyle (see pages 30–32). If the signs are that you are not ovulating, you may be referred for ovulation-stimulating treatment (see pages 150–51).

If your FSH level is high, there are measures you can take to try and bring it down (see pages 164–65), but bear in mind that, if the level is very high, you may be menopausal. Your doctor can refer you for ovulation-stimulating treatment. It may be that in vitro fertilization (IVF) is considered to be the best route, but you will have to wait until your FSH level has come down before you can start. If the level is high, you will not respond to treatment. The last route would be egg donation.

If prolactin levels are raised, a referral to an endocrinologist may be recommended. You will be checked for a pituitary tumour, and given medication to lower the levels (see page 130).

If thyroid-stimulating hormone (TSH) is high, further thyroid testing will be carried out to see whether you have an under-active thyroid.

If testosterone is high, further investigation will be required (fasting, blood-sugar test and insulin test) to check for PCOS.

As far as progesterone is concerned, if the result is less than 15, the blood test will be repeated during another menstrual cycle and, if it is still low, you will be referred to a fertility specialist. A result that is greater than 30 suggests that ovulation is adequate.

If all your hormonal levels appear to be normal and you are ovulating, further testing will be recommended to discover why you have been unable to conceive.

Raised levels of FSH

If your levels of FSH (follicle-stimulating hormone) are found to be high following a blood test, it is worth having the test repeated. Raised levels of FSH, depending on how high they are, may be a sign that you have a hormonal imbalance (see pages 30–32).

Ask your GP to do a full fertility check, along with an anti-mullerian hormone (AMH) blood test and antral follicle scan to check for any underlying issues.

Level two: tubal and uterine assessment

Once your hormones, and hence ovulation, have been checked, the next step is to look for blockages in your Fallopian tubes that could prevent the progress of egg or sperm, or uterine problems that might prevent implantation. Your doctor or fertility specialist will refer you to a hospital for these tests to determine whether or not there is a blockage and, if there is, its location in your reproductive system. These procedures are usually carried out during the first half of the cycle. Some clinics prescribe a course of antibiotics first to get rid of any infection.

The Fallopian tubes

Blocked tubes account for 20 per cent of female infertility. They can sometimes be unblocked surgically. Blockages may be caused by:

* **an infection,** perhaps a sexually transmitted one (see page 108)

* **pelvic inflammatory disease** (see page 108), which is caused by a sexually transmitted infection, the insertion of an intra-uterine device (IUD, or coil) or bacteria. It is a good idea for both you and your partner to be checked for STIs and to get immediate treatment if you are harbouring any infection

* **adhesions** (scar tissue) from previous surgery.

Hysterosalpingogram

This is a routine test, known as an HSG for short, that will identify blockage in the Fallopian tubes. A small tube is inserted into the cervix and liquid dye squirted through it. X-rays are taken as the dye enters the reproductive organs, picking up its course and showing up any obstructions, adhesions (scar tissue) or uterine abnormalities such as polyps (small growths that are usually harmless) or fibroids (see pages 117–19). You may experience temporary discomfort or cramping with this test, but the level of pain is variable.

Some studies indicate that the likelihood of pregnancy might increase slightly in the first few months following an HSG, possibly because flushing out the tubes removes minor blockages.

What next?

If there is a blockage in your Fallopian tubes, your specialist will recommend a laparoscopy (see below) to determine the nature and extent of the obstruction. Minor treatment of the tubes may be required. If there are no blockages, you may still need a laparoscopy or a hysteroscopy (see below) to check the uterine cavity.

Laparoscopy

This is an invasive test requiring a general anaesthetic and a short hospital admission. A tiny incision is made near your navel and the abdominal cavity is filled with carbon dioxide gas, which is intended to separate the organs and enable them to be seen better. A laparoscope, resembling a small telescope, is inserted so that the doctor can inspect the abdominal cavity, uterus and Fallopian tubes for anything unusual such as fibroids or endometriosis. The aftereffects of this procedure may include pain in the abdomen, neck or shoulders (caused by the gas) or vaginal bleeding.

Hysteroscopy

This may be done in some clinics at the same time as a laparoscopy. A hysteroscopy requires you to be mildly sedated or have a local anaesthetic. A viewing instrument called a hysteroscope is inserted via the cervix into the uterine cavity to check for irregularities or adhesions. This also allows for your uterus to be "mapped" for future reference, which in many clinics is part of the preparation for in vitro fertilization (IVF).

What next?

If you have fibroids, your specialist can determine their size and number, and assess whether they are likely to be affecting your fertility. You may receive treatment and may be able to return to Plan A. If endometriosis (see pages 114–16) is detected, treatment may enable you to return to Plan A.

Level three: immunological screening

This is specialist screening and will be recommended if you have a history of miscarriage or as yet unidentified fertility problems.

Blood screening can be done by your doctor, and indeed should have been suggested if you have suffered repeated miscarriage. Usually, two blood tests are carried out six weeks apart. Alternatively, you can be referred for this testing by an auto-immune specialist or at a fertility clinic, depending on your history, or it may be part of your doctor's initial investigations into your fertility.

Certain reactions instigated by the immune system may result in your body rejecting a fertilized embryo (see pages 124–25). Your fertility consultant may suggest immunological screening if there are no apparent reasons for your fertility problems after you have undergone hormone assessment or tubal and uterine investigative procedures and your partner has had sperm analysis or other tests.

Problems with the immune system are increasingly believed to be a significant factor in some cases of pregnancy loss. Numerous studies have discovered abnormal levels of particular antibodies in women who experience either IVF failure or repeated miscarriage and have otherwise found no cause of their fertility problems.

The immunological investigative process is a complex and expensive one and involves repeat testing throughout early pregnancy once you have conceived, but it may be worth considering by couples who:

* have had two or more miscarriages
* have unexplained infertility
* have good embryos that fail to implant during IVF procedures.

Dealing with antibodies

If you have consistently high levels of antiphospholipid or anticardiolipin antibodies, you will have about a 10–20 per cent chance of carrying a pregnancy. You may be given a low dose of aspirin a day to thin the blood. Heparin may also be offered. Thickened blood (as a result of the antibodies) increases the likelihood of miscarriage because it reduces blood flow through the placenta and increases the chance of blood clots, which have the same effect. The presence of anti-nuclear antibodies may well give rise to inflammation of the uterus. Inflammation of any kind in the pelvic region can put a foetus at risk. If these antibodies are detected, you may be given steroids to reduce inflammation.

If you have natural killer cells, any embryos will be rejected and therefore fail to implant. Possible treatment in this instance is highly controversial, not readily available, very expensive and carries with it other serious risks (see page 125) so you would need to research and consider this option very carefully indeed.

Natural killer cells are a type of white blood cell and part of the body's immune response mechanism.

Female fertility problems

A diagnosis can bring with it a great sense of relief. Now that you have identified the problem, you may feel encouraged by the fact that there are things you can do to alleviate it and maximize your chances of either natural or assisted conception.

Understanding a diagnosis

You may already be aware of a problem in your reproductive system – menstrual irregularities, for example – or perhaps you have just been diagnosed with a particular condition as a result of fertility tests. It is important to learn about your condition and appreciate its implications for your chances of conceiving a baby. You need to be able to recognize symptoms; understand the causes, if they are known; be aware of factors making you susceptible; learn how the condition is treated; and determine ways of improving your health and lifestyle to make a difference to your fertility.

Some conditions that diminish fertility are underlying general health issues; others are caused by infections; some are to do with the functioning of the reproductive cycle and system parts; while others are the result of physiological irregularities. They are all described in the following pages.

I would always recommend that you combine the advice of your conventional doctors with any of the many complementary treatments and remedies you might choose to try in order to improve your condition. And never underestimate the importance of good nutrition, too, in an integrated plan to improve your fertility.

Causes of fertility problems (UK)

		PRIMARY INFERTILITY	SECONDARY INFERTILITY
Primary infertility is when a couple have being trying for their first baby for a year or more but have been unsuccessful.	• ovulatory	20 per cent	15 per cent
	• tubal	15 per cent	40 per cent
Secondary infertility is when a couple have a child but have difficulty conceiving subsequently. A significant	• endometriosis	10 per cent	5 per cent
number of cases in each category are unattributable to any one cause. Figures vary	• male problems	25 per cent	20 per cent
from one clinic to another.	• unexplained	30 per cent	20 per cent

Underlying conditions

There are many conditions that are not directly related to the female reproductive system but have implications for a woman's fertility. Sometimes common conditions, such as anaemia and thyroid problems, may be overlooked.

Anaemia

Iron deficiency is one of the most common causes of anaemia. It is estimated that more than 50 per cent of women worldwide get less than the recommended intake of 10–15mg/day. It is much harder to conceive if you are anaemic and the body is, in effect, fighting on all fronts. Other types of anaemia include folic-acid deficiency and pernicious anaemia.

What is it? Every body cell needs oxygen, which is carried by the pigment haemoglobin in red blood cells. Anaemia results when there are too few red blood cells. It can take a long time to restore normal levels once they have fallen.

What are the symptoms?
Symptoms depend on the severity of the condition and include:
* shortness of breath
* dizziness and palpitations
* lethargy and weakness
* susceptibility to infection
* loss of appetite
* skin pallor
* heavy periods
* emotional fragility.

What causes it? Apart from too few iron-rich foods in the diet, factors limiting iron absorption include a high zinc intake; a lack of B vitamins; too much tea and coffee; a high wheat-bran intake; antacids that are taken for heartburn; and too many dairy products. Dairy-rich and iron-rich foods should be eaten separately.

Who is at risk? Women with malabsorption problems, such as coeliac disease, or heavy periods are prone. Frequent dieters and vegetarians are also at risk.

How is it diagnosed? A simple blood test. Haemoglobin levels in a healthy female should be 11–15.

How is it treated conventionally? Iron supplements are prescribed but are not easily absorbed. There are many on the market that have a gentle effect.

Can complementary therapies help? Specific acupoints can be treated by an acupuncturist to "build the blood".

Diet and nutrition

Iron, protein, copper, folic acid and vitamins B6, B12 and C are all necessary for the formation of red blood cells. A deficiency in any of these nutrients may cause anaemia. Make sure you eat lots of the following kinds of food:

* **Iron-rich foods** such as organ meats, lean meat, eggs, fish, poultry, molasses, cherries, apricots, dried fruits, green leafy vegetables, parsley, pumpkin and sunflower seeds, kelp, seaweed and nuts. Steep a large handful of the dried herb in hot water and drink 1–4 cups daily.

* **Foods rich in vitamin B12** which are principally animal products and especially lamb, sardines and salmon.

* **Foods rich in folic acid** such as dark-green leafy vegetables, organ meats, salmon, avocados, whole grains, pulses and dried figs.

* **Foods rich in vitamin C** – such as blackcurrants, kiwi fruit, citrus fruits, melon, mangos, pineapple, parsley, watercress and broccoli – which improve iron absorption.

Diabetes

There is no direct link between insulin-dependent diabetes and fertility, but high insulin levels in the blood and impaired glucose tolerance may result in an absence of ovulation. Those with uncontrolled diabetes are six times more likely to miscarry.

What is it? This is a metabolic disorder; the pancreas fails to secrete enough insulin to help cells to absorb glucose for energy.

What are the symptoms? They may go unnoticed until you have a medical check-up. They are:

* lack of energy
* blurred vision
* excessive urination
* recurrent thrush
* thirst and a dry mouth.

What causes it? Diabetes occurs most commonly when body cells become resistant to insulin.

Who is at risk? You are more at risk if diabetes runs in your family or you are obese.

How is it diagnosed? A simple test checks for the presence of sugar in the urine or blood.

Diet and nutrition

In women, diabetes is often associated with being **overweight.** Be guided by your doctor, who may refer you to a dietician for help with the condition and control of your weight. Abnormal metabolic reactions tend to generate many free radicals so make sure you take **antioxidant supplements** (see pages 59–61).

How is it treated? Mild diabetes can be controlled by means of dietary measures alone, but more severe cases require regular insulin injections to control blood-sugar levels.

Diet and nutrition

A nutritional therapist can help you work out a **dietary programme for managing an under-active thyroid** (but only in conjunction with conventional medicine). Essential nutrients are needed to ensure that there are no "gaps" in the metabolic pathways and energy production is not impaired. Make sure you get enough of the following **essential nutrients** (see pages 59–64):

* vitamins B1, B2, B3, B5 and B6
* co-enzyme Q10
* magnesium
* chromium
* selenium
* zinc
* iodine
* calcium.

Under-active thyroid

Thyroid hormones control the speed of metabolic processes so the body has enough energy to drive all its systems, including those that are part of reproduction. They also increase protein synthesis for the maintenance and repair of the body and are therefore extremely important for every body cell.

Thyroxine (T4) is the main thyroid hormone, but it is inactive physiologically and has to be converted into an active form – T3 (triiodothyronine) – to do its job.

What is it? Underlying thyroid dysfunction affects the frequency of ovulation and may even prevent it altogether (anovulation). A shortage of thyroid hormones is known as hypothyroidism. Thyroid dysfunction is commonly found to be a contributory factor in female fertility problems today.

What are the symptoms? Symptoms of an under-active thyroid vary from person to person and may be mild or debilitating. Everyone has their own physical strengths and weaknesses, depending on genetic make-up, diet and lifestyle. As energy is depleted as a result of thyroid dysfunction, an individual's most vulnerable systems will suffer first. Symptoms may include:

* weakness and exhaustion
* memory impairment
* dry hair or hair loss
* sensitivity to cold
* skin problems and
  brittle nails
* depression and mood swings
* constipation
* weight gain or weight loss
* heavy or irregular periods
* PMS (premenstrual syndrome)
* muscle cramps and joint stiffness.

What causes it? There are three main causes of this condition:
* failure of the thyroid gland itself
* failure of the feedback mechanisms that prompt the thyroid gland to secrete more hormones
* failure of body tissues to use thyroid hormones properly.

Who is at risk? Women are generally affected more than men, especially those who have experienced substantial weight loss or who have a history of thyroid disorders in the family.

How is it diagnosed? Often a simple blood test. A TSH (thyroid-stimulating hormone) level that is beyond the expected range, combined with a level of thyroxine (T_4) that is below the expected range or even within it, usually indicates an under-active thyroid.

You may also be told you have tested positive for thyroid antibodies, which can be present without thyroid dysfunction and therefore remain undiagnosed. Your doctor will advise you on the most appropriate form of treatment.

How is it treated conventionally? A daily dose of synthetic thyroxine hormone is the drug prescribed. Conventional treatment is essential.

Can complementary therapies help? Complementary therapies cannot tackle hormone imbalance directly. Hypothyroidism is a complex disorder that must be treated with conventional medicine. Dietary measures include the intake of essential nutrients (see box, opposite). Regular gentle exercise and other lifestyle changes may be helpful as part of a holistic thyroid treatment plan.

Acupuncture may help to encourage thyroid function as part of the harmonious functioning of the body as a whole, but complementary therapies should never be substituted for prescribed drugs to treat the problem.

Zita's tips

Indicators of thyroid issues, a contributory factor in female fertility problems, are varied. As the symptoms can develop slowly, you may not realise that you have a medical problem for several years, so it can often remain undiagnosed. The following indicators may identify a thyroid problem:

* **Weight gain** but with a poor appetite. It is common to attribute weight gain to a reduction in activity levels or an increase in calorie intake, but it can sometimes be a potential sign of an underlying thyroid problem.

* **Irregular cycles** and excessive menstrual bleeding. Irregularities in your menstrual cycle, ranging from absent and infrequent periods to very frequent and heavy, can indicate thyroid issues.

* **Feeling exhausted,** sluggish and fatigued, even after having had proper rest, as your bodily functions slow down.

* **If you have suffered recurrent miscarriage,** talk to your doctor about thyroid screening.

* **Bowel problems.** You may suffer chronic constipation.

* **Muscle** aches and pains, cramps and general muscle weakness.

* **If you know you have a history** of thyroid problems in your family, speak to your doctor about screening.

Pelvic disorders

Any disorders of the female reproductive system may ultimately affect a woman's fertility, including pelvic infections, which are very common. If you think you may have an infection, get it checked out as soon as possible.

Pelvic inflammatory disease (PID)

Many women may have had PID in the past without knowing it because of a lack of symptoms. Long-standing or serious infection may cause scar tissue to build up around a Fallopian tube, preventing the passage of an egg. Ectopic pregnancy or miscarriage may also occur as a result.

What is it? PID is an umbrella term for any inflammation of the pelvic organs. Since there are often no symptoms, it is not known how many women are affected.

What are the symptoms? Many women are unaware they have PID until they start trying to conceive a baby. When there are symptoms, they can be acute or chronic and include:

* foul-smelling vaginal discharge
* fever, chills and nausea
* pain in the lower abdomen
* bleeding between periods
* painful intercourse
* a need to pass urine more frequently than usual
* painful urination.

What causes it? PID is usually the result of a chlamydial infection (see page 110) or another sexually transmitted infection (STI), such as gonorrhoea (see pages 110–11), spreading upwards from the vagina to the uterus and tubes.

Who is at risk? Women (or their partners) who have had a number of different sexual partners are at most risk from pelvic infections.

How is it diagnosed? A swab can be taken at an STI (sexually transmitted infections) clinic in your local hospital and analysed.

How is it treated conventionally? Antibiotics treat the infection; surgery can remove scar tissue.

Self-help measures include: dietary measures to fight infection (see page 111) and complementary remedies to aid the reproductive system (see pages 145–49).

Genito-urinary problems

Fertility is easily compromised by inflammation and other consequences of genito-urinary problems. Studies at one infertility clinic in the UK found that 69 per cent of their patients suffered from GU infections.

Certain pelvic infections in women can lead to PID (see above), blocked tubes, ectopic pregnancy and early miscarriage, and in men to damaged sperm and blocked ducts in the testes. If you or your partner have had a number of sexual partners, it is a good idea to get a sexual health screening to make sure you have no sexually transmitted infections (STIs). If either of you has, then you must both get treatment. Some STIs have a direct effect on fertility (see below). They can be bacterial, viral or mycoplasmal in origin. Other conditions, such as hepatitis, are passed on during intercourse and affect general health, which in turn impacts on fertility.

Many women today receive abnormal smear-test results as a result of cervical dysplasia. This may have a number of causes. Any treatment required may lengthen the time it takes to conceive.

Candida (Dysbiosis)

Any condition that compromises your general state of health and leads to nutritional imbalances can have a negative effect on fertility. An overgrowth of certain micro-organisms in the vagina may make intercourse painful and create a hostile environment for sperm.

What is it? *Candida albicans* is a yeast that occurs naturally in the gut, on the skin and in the vagina as part of a network of micro-organisms keeping the body healthy. If the candida yeast proliferates, dysbiosis, more commonly known as candida or candidiasis, may result. It is a very common complaint.

What causes it? Candida is usually kept under control by "friendly" bacteria in the gut. In certain circumstances, however, the good bacteria are compromised and candida organisms proliferate.

Who is at risk? Several factors may contribute to a proliferation of candida:
* poor nutrition
* a diet high in refined sugars
* taking broad-spectrum antibiotics
* long-term use of steroids
* surgery, especially gastrointestinal
* disease or illness
* stress
* hormone imbalance with an excess of oestrogen
* poor adrenal function.

What are the symptoms? There are many symptoms associated with this condition and often there aren't any obvious or separate characteristics. They may include:
* food cravings, especially sugars
* bloating and flatulence
* vaginitis or cystitis
* vaginal thrush
* changes in bowel habits
* irritable bowel syndrome (IBS)
* depression or lethargy
* impaired absorption of nutrients
* alcohol intolerance.

How is it diagnosed? Testing for candida overgrowth is not easy,

Zita's tips

* **Buy a good probiotic supplement** (*Lactobacillus acidophilus*) to re-colonize the gut with beneficial flora.

* **Eat a daily portion** of "live" yoghurt containing *Lactobacillus acidophilus*.

* **Wear loose-fitting cotton** underwear to promote a cooler, less moist environment.

* **Avoid using bubble bath;** put a handful of salt in the bath water or a few drops of anti-fungal tea tree oil.

* **If candida varies in degree** try a candida diet, but this will need to be supervised.

Diet and nutrition

Diet is probably the best way to deal with candida, both as a preventative measure and as a cure. A completely sugar-free diet is almost impossible to achieve, but try cutting back on foods that can contribute to candida overgrowth:

* **cut out refined sugars and** natural sweeteners such as honey and maple syrup

* **avoid alcohol** as it is high in sugar that can feed the growth of the candida yeast.

You may notice that symptoms initially get worse before they improve, as a reaction to candida die-off (dead yeast organisms).

and there is great debate among medical practitioners about its efficacy. Some believe there has been a tendency for complementary health practitioners to diagnose this condition too readily.

How is it treated conventionally? Candida is usually treated with anti-fungal creams and pessaries; these can be applied to any affected areas.

Can complementary therapies help? Many people benefit from an anti-fungal and anti-candida diet (see box, above). Constitutional homeopathic treatment may also be helpful.

Chlamydia

Tubal damage caused by acute inflammation of the Fallopian tubes (salpingitis) or other forms of pelvic inflammatory disease (PID, see page 108) is the most common cause of female infertility. Research suggests that as many as 66 per cent of cases of salpingitis and 30 per cent of other pelvic inflammatory diseases are caused by *Chlamydia trachomatis*. Some women suffer little, if at all, as a result of having this bacterial infection, while others experience extensive damage to their reproductive systems – with long-term implications for fertility – from a minimal level of infection.

What is it? A micro-organism found in the genito-urinary tract, chlamydia causes mild to severe infection. Believed to be the most common sexually transmitted, disease-carrying organism in the Western world, it infects the cervix first, causing chlamydial cervicitis, then spreads to the endometrium. If left untreated, it can move into the Fallopian tubes, causing acute salpingitis or PID. Chlamydia is now a widespread complaint: as many as 15–20 per cent of sexually active people show evidence of previous chlamydial infection, and the number of reported cases is on the increase.

What are the symptoms?
You may develop a slight vaginal discharge for a couple of weeks, but if the infection attacks the cervix, there may be no outward indications at all. Chlamydia is known as a "silent infection" because of this: it has been estimated that more than 70 per cent of infected women exhibit no symptoms at all.

Who is at risk? Women are at greater risk of having contracted this disease if they have had a number of sexual partners. The UK government is actively pursuing the idea of a national chlamydia screening programme (based on urine tests), but there are many issues to be resolved before this becomes a reality.

How is it diagnosed? A swab is taken from the cells of the cervix to identify any infection. A hysterosalpingogram (see page 102) will reveal the extent of any tubal damage. Both partners should be tested for infection.

How is it treated conventionally?
Antibiotics – usually a 10–14 day course of treatment – almost guarantee a cure. It is advisable to use a condom during sexual intercourse to protect you from any further infection.

Self-help measures include:
nutrition and dietary measures to help fight infection (see opposite).

Gonorrhoea

It is estimated that about 1 million people in the US alone become infected with gonorrhoea each year. The disease is much less widespread than it used to be, however, as a result of early detection, improved methods of treatment and safe-sex practices, but it is still one of the most common STIs. Twice as many men as women are infected.

Early treatment of this sexually transmitted infection is crucially important: if it is detected almost immediately, there is little chance of lasting damage. Undetected infection in women, however, can spread up through the uterus, eventually infecting and damaging

Gonorrhoea bacteria (red) are surrounding other cells (green) in this image.

the Fallopian tubes, causing them to become misshapen and blocked. In addition, untreated gonorrhoea increases a woman's chances of an ectopic pregnancy.

What is it? A bacterial infection (*Neisseria gonorrhoeae*), gonorrhoea is one of the most infectious diseases there is. It is one of the major causes of pelvic inflammatory disease (PID) and leaves women more susceptible to contracting chlamydial infections.

What are the symptoms? Within five days of intercourse with an infected partner, a man will have a creamy discharge from the urethra and it may hurt to pass urine. Abdominal pain and high fever will follow. A woman may have similar symptoms, but more than 70 per cent of infected women exhibit no symptoms at all.

Who is at risk? Unprotected sex with many different partners will put you at increased risk.

How is it diagnosed? A swab is taken from the infected area and tested for the bacteria. Both partners should be tested.

How is it treated conventionally? Penicillin effectively kills the bacteria and the infection should clear up within four or five days, but you should be retested about 10 days after treatment to make sure you are clear of infection before having sex again.

Helping fight infection

Boosting the immune system by eating a nutrient-rich diet and taking a good multivitamin and mineral supplement is the best way of preventing infections from spreading. Eliminate foods containing yeast and sugar to help fight yeast infection.

If you are on antibiotics, take a probiotic (disease-destroying bacteria) supplement, such as *Lactobacillus acidophilus* (three capsules a day usually) or eat a small pot of live yoghurt that contains "active" bacterial cultures. Other supplements known to be helpful for vaginal infections include:

* **Vitamin C** – helps the formation of collagen. If the collagen matrix (the main component of the body's connective tissue) is intact, infection will be less able to spread, you will develop less scar tissue and damaged tissue will repair more quickly.
* **Betacarotene** – a powerful antioxidant that is vital for the functioning of the immune system and the normal growth of vaginal tissue. It also helps to fight infection.
* **Vitamin E** – increases resistance to chlamydial infections. As well as taking it orally, you can open a capsule and apply the oil directly to the inflamed area to soothe and heal. Yeast-free capsules may also be inserted into the vagina.

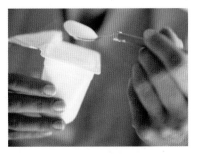

Eat a portion of live yoghurt every day to help restore "friendly" bacteria in the gut and vagina.

* **B vitamins** – needed to fight infection. Women with vaginal infections are very often found to be deficient in B vitamins.
* **Vitamin D** – important for a number of functions in the body and boosting immunity.
* **Zinc** – boosts immunity, encourages healing and prevents recurrence of infection.
* **Garlic** – has strong antibacterial properties to help fight infection.
* *Lactobacillus acidophilus* supplement (with at least 4 billion beneficial bacteria) – this is antagonistic to unfriendly bacteria and toxic to *Gardnerella vaginalis*, the bacteria responsible for many infections of the vagina and vulva. Usually taken orally, but may be inserted into the vagina.

Herpes

This condition is widespread. Many people who have it are reluctant to talk about it, however.

What is it? Genital herpes is closely related to herpes type 1, which causes cold sores on the lips. The virus can lie dormant for years before the first outbreak.

What are the symptoms? A burning sensation on the labia is followed by itching and a crop of small blisters. These crust over and heal in about a week, but you might be infectious for another five days.

What causes it? After the initial attack, the virus lies dormant rather than disappearing, although the body produces antibodies that help prevent further attacks. The virus may be reactivated by stress, menstruation, depression, anxiety, a suppressed immune system, lack of sleep or poor diet. Outbreaks occur less frequently over time.

Who is at risk? Those having unprotected sex with multiple partners are most at risk.

How is it diagnosed? A swab taken from an active herpetic sore can be analysed, or a blood test may identify herpes antibodies.

How is it treated conventionally? An anaesthetic ointment and some pain relief is usually prescribed.

The drug acyclovir (Zovirax) may reduce the severity of symptoms if applied early enough.

Can complementary therapies help? Acupuncture may help to boost the immune system, for example, but conventional drugs are needed to treat the infection.

Self-help measures include:
* avoiding sex during an attack
* taking multivitamins and minerals, especially vitamin C, bioflavonoids and zinc
* avoiding arginine-rich foods
* applying tea-tree oil or calendula ointment to the blisters
* exposing the area to the air
* taking garlic capsules at onset.

Bacterial vaginosis

Studies have shown that couples with fertility problems are more likely than fertile couples to have high concentrations of some of the minute micro-organisms that normally inhabit the genital tract. These include *Gardnerella vaginalis, Mycoplasma hominis, Ureaplasma urealyticum* and Group B *Streptococcus*.

What is it? Although some of these are the smallest disease-carrying organisms, if they are allowed to proliferate, the balance between all the micro-organisms in the genital tract is altered, causing a variety of genito-urinary problems, especially if your general health is poor and the immune system is weakened. Rarely, women may go on to develop pelvic inflammatory disease (PID, see page 108).

What are the symptoms? There may not be any, but some women experience a vaginal discharge or vulvovaginitis – inflammation of the vagina and vulva.

What causes it? The reasons for overgrowth of organisms are not fully understood, but the condition may be associated with another sexually transmitted infection.

Who is at risk? Those having unprotected sex with multiple partners are most at risk.

How is it diagnosed? Bacterial vaginosis may be obvious from the symptoms, but a swab will often be taken to confirm the diagnosis. Both partners should be checked.

How is it treated conventionally? A course of antibiotics will clear up the infection within a couple of days, but the condition does tend to recur.

Self-help measures include: nutrition and dietary measures to help fight infection (see page 111).

Can complementary therapies help? Complementary therapies may help to boost the immune system and help fight infection.

Reproductive organ dysfunctions

Problems with the basic functioning of the female reproductive system range from physical problems in parts of the reproductive organs to malfunctions of the processes of egg production, fertilization, implantation and development.

Ectopic pregnancy

This is an implantation problem: a fertilized egg does not implant in the lining of the uterus but in tissue outside it. The egg then begins to develop into an embryo, but it is not able to grow normally and will never survive.

What is it? An ectopic pregnancy develops outside the uterus, usually in one of the Fallopian tubes. About one in 100 pregnancies is ectopic.

What are the symptoms? Common signs include:
* abdominal pain, often on one side
* vaginal bleeding, often with dark blood, "like prune juice"
* a missed period and symptoms of pregnancy
* faintness and light-headedness
* shoulder pain (referred pain).

What causes it? Damage to a Fallopian tube may restrict the passage of an egg to the uterus, but the cause is not always known.

Who is at risk? There is an increased risk of having an ectopic pregnancy if you have:

* previously had a pelvic infection
* had surgery on the Fallopian tubes or ovaries
* had a previous ectopic pregnancy, which increases the risk of having another one 20-fold
* used an intra-uterine device (IUD, or coil) as a contraceptive
* had in vitro fertilization (IVF) treatment.

How is it diagnosed? As well as a pregnancy and blood test, you may be referred for:
* an ultrasound scan
* a laparoscopy (see page 102).

How is it treated conventionally? An ectopic pregnancy is usually dealt with surgically as soon as possible. The tube is opened up, the embryo removed and the tube repaired using keyhole surgery, or, if it is badly damaged, removed altogether. A larger cut above the pubic hairline may be necessary if the pregnancy needs to be dealt with urgently or if keyhole surgery is not possible.

Following an ectopic pregnancy, there is a higher risk of another one in subsequent pregnancies. It

Case history

Tara, aged 32, conceived within a few months, but soon developed spotting and pain. A scan revealed an ectopic pregnancy and evidence of a previous pelvic infection. Tara did not want to go straight to IVF (in vitro fertilization). Despite there still being a risk of an ectopic pregnancy because of tubal scarring, she opted to improve her diet for six months before trying again. If she had no success, she would then try IVF.

is advisable to have an early scan to ensure that implantation is in the uterus. Your fertility may be slightly reduced by having a Fallopian tube removed, but most women conceive and deliver subsequently with no complications.

Diet and nutrition

Good nutrition is vitally important in treating the underlying causes of endometriosis. (Consider a detox programme – see pages 50–53.)

To help balance oestrogen levels:

* increase your intake of dietary fibre, especially whole grains, pulses, brown rice, flax seeds, fruits and vegetables
* eat bitter foods such as chicory and radicchio, and vegetables such as cabbage, cauliflower, Brussels sprouts, broccoli and turnips, to aid oestrogen clearance via the bowel
* reduce your saturated fat intake and cut down on meat and dairy produce
* avoid foods containing sugar, chocolate, caffeine and alcohol
* eat foods containing natural phyto-oestrogens (see page 31)

To help reduce inflammation:

* eat fruits rich in vitamin C and bioflavonoids, especially the pulp and inner peel of citrus fruits, grape skins and berries
* take a daily multivitamin and mineral supplement containing vitamins B-complex, C and E, zinc, magnesium, and selenium (see pages 59–63)
* take a daily supplement of omega-3 essential fatty acids and evening primrose oil (see also pages 63–64)
* avoid partially hydrogenated oils, including margarine.

Endometriosis

A large number of women who undergo a laparoscopic procedure (see page 102) to investigate the possible causes of their fertility problems are found to be suffering from endometriosis. This condition is not the direct cause of infertility but it may be a major contributory factor. The root cause of it may also be responsible for the woman's failure to conceive.

If the extent is mild-moderate to severe and there are adhesions (scar tissue) and tubal and/or ovarian damage, ovulation and fertilization will obviously be affected. If the condition is mild, with only a few scattered implants, the link with infertility is more difficult to establish. It may be because more prostaglandins (hormone-like substances) are produced in the pelvic cavity. These may interfere with ovulation and affect the muscles in the Fallopian tubes, preventing transportation of the egg along the tube. It may be because there is an increased number of white blood cells attacking and destroying foreign bodies, including sperm or embryos. Tackling the underlying causes of endometriosis is therefore perhaps the best option.

What is it? The migration and implantation of endometrial tissue, which forms the lining of the uterus, in other parts of the body, usually in the pelvic region (ovaries, Fallopian tubes, uterine muscles, colon and bladder) but occasionally outside it. These "implants" are stimulated by hormonal changes, so they build up and then bleed in the same way as the lining of the uterus does, causing scarring and adhesions.

Estimates of how common a complaint this is range from 4–17 per cent of all menstruating females, but the figure could be higher. Endometriosis is believed to be the cause of as much as 80 per cent of pelvic pain.

What are the symptoms? The severity of symptoms is not related to the severity of the condition. You may have no symptoms or a combination of several, including:

* severe pain or cramp in the pelvis, abdomen, leg or lower back
* pain during bowel movements or urination
* pain during intercourse
* abnormal menstruation
* spotting between periods
* heavy bleeding with thick clots
* severe premenstrual syndrome (PMS – see pages 126–27) with bloating, sore breasts, cravings and headaches
* mood swings, anxiety, irritability, depression, and a feeling of being overwhelmed
* fatigue, exhaustion and low energy levels.

What causes it? The cause is not known but there are a number of theories. It is probably due to a

combination of factors, including:
* excess oestrogen (see pages 31–32)
* menstruation starting at an early age or delayed pregnancy
* retrograde menstruation, whereby blood and tissue flow backwards into the Fallopian tubes
* a weakness that some women have in their pelvic area, making them vulnerable to infections and conditions such as candida overgrowth (see page 109)
* a weakened immune system (as a result of chronic stress, poor diet, nutritional deficiencies, etc.).
In Traditional Chinese Medicine (see page 72), endometriosis is believed to be the result of a blockage in or "stagnation" of the flow of energy around the body.

Who is at risk? Several factors may combine to increase the risk of endometriosis, including:
* regular heavy periods that last more than seven days
* an immediate family member – a mother or a sister – who has endometriosis
* strenuous physical activity while menstruating (although regular exercise reduces the risk)
* using an intra-uterine device (IUD), which may increase the amount of retrograde blood flow.

How is it diagnosed? If your medical history reveals a number of symptoms usually associated with endometriosis, you will be given a pelvic examination. Depending on the findings, you may then be referred to a specialist gynaecology clinic for an ultrasound scan. This uses high-frequency sound waves to create images of the pelvic cavity so that abnormalities may be spotted. Alternatively, you may have a laparoscopy (see page 102), which is the best means of confirming a diagnosis of endometriosis.

How is it treated conventionally?
Conventional Western medicine uses the following methods:
* painkillers
* synthetic hormones, usually the contraceptive pill,

Ultrasound scanning allows your specialist to "see" into the pelvic cavity. It can be used to diagnose endometriosis.

Zita's tips

* **Take regular exercise**, especially first thing in the morning, and avoid strenuous activity during a period.

* **Make sure you take** plenty of rest when you need to.

* **Use painkillers**, but try to cut down on using analgesic drugs altogether.

* **Relax in an Epsom-salt bath** to relax the muscles deeply and release emotions and stress. Dissolve a tub of salts in hot water and immerse yourself for 20 minutes or so. When you are dry, lie down quietly for another 20 minutes.

* **Do not use tampons** or, if you must, make sure they are 100 per cent cotton. In Chinese medicine, tampons are believed to interfere with the free flow of blood from the body.

synthetic progesterone or gonadotrophin-releasing hormone (GnRH) to arrest the further development of endometrial lesions

* surgery: the laparoscopic removal of lesions or small cysts from the endometrium may be possible (see page 102), but sometimes microsurgery will be necessary to remove adhesions from less accessible locations within the pelvic cavity or Fallopian tubes. Laser surgery may also be used (during a laparoscopic procedure) to destroy small areas of endometrial tissue, increasing your chances of conception for about 4–6 months until the condition recurs.

Can complementary therapies help? A combination of dietary and lifestyle changes together with specific complementary treatments can be used to tackle the underlying causes of the condition, reduce the severity of the symptoms and minimize the chances of recurrence. Every individual is different, so you need to work out the right programme for you with the help of a complementary practitioner. Treatments to try include:

* herbal remedies, such as chaste-tree berry (*Vitex agnus castus*) to encourage ovulation
* acupuncture, to restore balance between the body's systems, improve the flow of vital energy and relieve pain
* homeopathy: constitutional remedies recommended might include cimicifuga, coffea or folliculinum, depending on your particular symptoms.

Case history

*Rosy, aged 38, used the Billings method of natural contraception for four years before actively trying to conceive. After eight months without success she visited a gynaecologist who diagnosed severe (grade 2) endometriosis. Rosy had always suffered very heavy, painful periods with a lot of clotting, but she had taken this for granted as "normal" for her. **After reading an article by a fellow endometriosis sufferer, she cut out wheat, dairy products and caffeine from her diet.** Although this was not easy to do, she was very determined and noticed an improvement almost immediately: her next period was lighter and less painful. **On the recommendation** of a friend, she started coming to me for acupuncture. After weekly treatments throughout one cycle, Rosy conceived her daughter Agnes, who is 16 months old at the time of writing.*

*Rosy breastfed Agnes for ten months, during which time she had no periods. **Two months after her periods resumed, she discovered she was pregnant again.** Sadly, she miscarried this baby at 13 weeks. During both pregnancies she says she "never felt healthier".*

She has been advised to try to conceive another baby as soon as possible because of her age. She has been taking a preconceptual multivitamin and mineral supplement for many months, follows a healthy diet and avoids alcohol.

Fibroids

Fibroids growing on the walls of the uterus won't necessarily stop you getting pregnant, but even very small fibroids can interfere with endometrial development and implantation (see page 12). Fibroids any larger than about 4–5cm (1½–2in) in diameter may cause problems during pregnancy as they push against blood vessels, possibly preventing the foetus from developing normally.

Some fibroids grow outside the uterus but, if they are larger than 6cm (2½in) in diameter, they may get in the way as the Fallopian tube tries to pick up an egg after ovulation, and this could affect your ability to conceive. However, once you are pregnant, small fibroids will not hurt your developing baby. Many women go to term without their fibroids causing any problems.

What are they? Fibroids are benign tumours that grow in the uterine cavity, in the muscular walls of the uterus or on the outside of the uterus. Only very rarely, in less than 0.5 per cent of cases, do they become malignant. Fibroids vary enormously in size, from microscopic to the size of a football, and are made of a hard, white, gristly tissue. Their size often fluctuates during the menstrual cycle, growing after ovulation and shrinking after a period, according to hormonal changes. They usually shrink rapidly after menopause. Fibroids are the most common structural abnormalities of the uterus, and it is estimated that between 20–50 per cent of women aged from 35–50 have them. They are more common in black women than Caucasians, although it is not understood why.

What are the symptoms? It depends on the size and location of the fibroids, but many women have no symptoms at all and may be quite unaware that they have them. Possible symptoms caused by large fibroids include:
* heavy or irregular bleeding if the fibroids are growing in the uterine lining
* menstrual cramps and/or pelvic pain, if there is also endometriosis present
* extremely heavy bleeding, almost haemorrhaging, leaving you exhausted and anaemic
* pain, if the fibroid has outgrown its blood supply and started to degenerate, in which case the nerve at the centre of the fibroid registers the lack of oxygen as pain. As the fibroid shrinks and the nerve adjusts, the pain usually decreases
* a feeling of fullness or pressure in the lower abdomen, if the fibroid is quite large and is pressing on internal organs
* constipation
* the need to pass water frequently and urgently,

Diet and nutrition

Fibroids are oestrogen-sensitive, so a high-fat, high-protein, low-fibre diet will put you at greater risk of developing this condition, or exacerbating it, because more oestrogen will be circulating in the body as a result of eating these types of food. Changing to a low-fat, high-fibre, mostly vegetarian diet for at least three months may help to reduce the pain and bleeding associated with this condition.

* **Eliminate refined sugars,** wheat products, saturated fats, dairy products, chocolate, caffeine and salt from your diet as much as you can.

* **Include large quantities of** green leafy vegetables (such as spinach) and cruciferous vegetables (such as cauliflower and broccoli), whole grains (excluding wheat) and pulses.

* **Cut down on** red meat, poultry and alcohol.

* **Take an iron supplement** daily to prevent or relieve anaemia if you have heavy bleeding, together with a high dose of vitamin C and bioflavonoids to enhance iron absorption (see pages 57 and 61).

* **Take a good multivitamin and mineral supplement daily:** of particular importance are vitamin B-complex (especially its choline and inositol components), vitamin E, calcium, magnesium, potassium and the amino acid methionine (see pages 59–64).

Zita's tips

* **Take regular aerobic exercise**, such as swimming, cycling or running for at least 20 minutes three times a week.

* **Practise yoga** to reduce pelvic congestion, improve blood circulation, relax the muscles of the uterus and relax you generally, as well as improving your sense of wellbeing.

* **Use stress-reduction techniques** such as meditation, deep breathing, aromatherapy and massage (see pages 42–43).

* **Try herbal formulas** containing chaste-tree berry (*Vitex agnus castus*), dong quai, wild yam, liquorice root and sarsaparilla (see page 31), for example, but always make sure that you consult a qualified herbal practitioner before taking any herbal remedies.

* **Avoid using tampons** (see page 39) which hamper the free flow of blood from the body.

especially during the night, because the fibroid is exerting pressure on the bladder

* recurrent bladder infections or irritation.

What causes them? The cause is unknown.

Who is at risk? The following factors may increase your risk of developing fibroids.

* If a close female relative (your mother or a sister) has fibroids, it may mean you have a genetic predisposition to the condition, but dietary and environmental factors are believed to be more significant.

* A high-fat, low-fibre diet which encourages the circulation of oestrogen and contributes to constipation, which prevents the elimination of oestrogen.

* Obesity, possibly because of the production of non-ovarian oestrogen in fatty tissue.

How are they diagnosed? Fibroids are often detected in the first place during a routine pelvic examination. If they are growing inside the uterus, the diagnosis can be confirmed by means of an ultrasound scan. If they are located on the outer surface of the uterus, they will also be revealed on a scan or during a laparoscopic procedure (see page 102).

How are they treated conventionally? There are various methods of treatment, depending on the seriousness of the condition.

* If the fibroids aren't causing any problems, a wait-and-see policy may be adopted.

* Hormone therapy (synthetic or natural progesterone or gonadotrophin-releasing hormone – GnRH) may be prescribed to reduce levels of oestrogen and control bleeding, inducing temporary menopause.

Treatment of the appropriate reflex points may help to relieve pain and discomfort caused by changes to fibroids during your cycle.

* Fibroids can be surgically removed (myomectomy), usually by means of a hysteroscopic procedure (see page 102) via the cervix or by making an incision in the abdomen. Embolization (or uterine artery embolization procedure, to give it its full name) is a relatively new method of treating fibroids that is based on the principle of blocking off the supply of blood to a fibroid. This is, however, still regarded as being in the experimental stage, and is probably not suitable for those women with fibroids who are intending to have children.

Can complementary therapies help? Several therapies may help women with fibroids, either alone or in combination, by relieving the symptoms of excessive bleeding and pain and helping to reduce the size of fibroids so that myomectomy becomes a practical option. Complementary therapies may also help to tackle underlying causes of fibroids, especially the energetic and emotional patterns contributing to their development.

* Acupuncture, including moxabustion, can release blocked energy in the liver and pelvic area as well as relieving pain.

* Homeopathy may be helpful at a constitutional level to resolve both physiological and any emotional problems associated with this condition.
* Herbal remedies may help to reduce the size of fibroids and redress hormonal imbalance.
* Shiatsu or massage can increase the flow of life energy to the pelvic region.
* Reflexology, particularly on the reflex points for the uterus and liver, can release blocked energy.
* Counselling or psychotherapy can help you deal with underlying emotional issues that might be aggravating your state of health.

Polycystic ovary syndrome (PCOS)

PCOS is responsible for many of the fertility problems in the women I see. The underlying cause is the inability of the ovaries to produce hormones in the correct relative proportions. In addition, abnormally high levels of insulin may reduce egg quality. Women with PCOS tend to produce many small follicles, so there is an added risk of ovarian hyperstimulation syndrome (OHSS) if these women choose to go down the IVF (in vitro fertilization) route.

What is it? PCOS is a chronic condition in which the ovaries develop lots of tiny cysts just beneath the surface, caused by egg follicles that haven't matured properly. It is accompanied by hormonal imbalance and a variety of other characteristics such as a low level of progesterone and a high level of luteinizing hormone (LH). These abnormalities in hormone levels make it much more difficult for eggs to mature and to be released. Using non-steroidal anti-inflammatory drugs, such as ibuprofen and adult-strength aspirin, may contribute to the occurrence of PCOS.

It is estimated that 20 per cent of women have a tendency to polycystic ovaries, while 5–10 per cent have full-blown PCOS.

What are the symptoms? Symptoms often begin during adolescence or a woman's early 20s. They vary in severity and may include:

Diet and nutrition

Eating a **nutrient-rich, low-carb diet** will help your body to restore **hormonal balance.** Cut down on animal fats but increase amounts of **essential fatty acids.** Replace processed foods with **wholefoods.** Eat plenty of **vegetables and fruits,** preferably organic. Take a good multivitamin and mineral supplement.

* irregular or absent periods
* the absence of ovulation
* fertility problems or recurrent miscarriage
* rapid weight gain or difficulty losing weight
* increased amounts of facial hair, caused by the overproduction of androgens as well as raised levels of testosterone

Acupuncture

More research has been carried out into the effectiveness of acupuncture in the treatment of PCOS than for any other female reproductive problem. It includes **auricular acupuncture** (which uses acupoints located on the ear) and **electro-acupuncture,** whereby a low-intensity pulsing electric current is applied through the needles to stimulate acupoints. Acupuncture has long been recommended for improving cycle irregularities and relieving pain.

Acupuncture treatment impacts on B-endorphins, which in turn affect levels of gonadotrophin-releasing hormone (GnRH), and has been used in an attempt to regulate hormonal imbalance and specifically to adjust FSH and LH levels.

* skin problems such as acne or oily skin
* thinning hair or male-pattern hair loss
* insulin insensitivity leading to raised blood-sugar levels.

What causes it? PCOS is caused by a hormonal imbalance – an over-production of luteinizing hormone (LH), androgens or oestrogen, and an under-production of follicle-stimulating hormone (FSH) or progesterone. It is not known, however, whether the problem originates in the hypothalamus or the ovaries. Sometimes only one ovary is affected, which would suggest that the problem is ovarian.

Who is at risk? You are more at risk if you:
* are overweight or obese
* are a smoker

* have a family history of diabetes
* have close female relatives with the condition, which would suggest a genetic link.

How is it diagnosed? On an ultrasound scan the ovaries will appear enlarged because of multiple small cysts formed from undeveloped eggs. A blood test will detect hormonal imbalances (raised LH and low FSH levels). Blood pressure and blood-sugar levels should also be checked.

Self-testing is possible but results are unreliable because high levels of LH sometimes give a false positive in an ovulation-kit test. Your BTM (basal temperature measurement) may be erratic and difficult to determine accurately.

How is it treated conventionally? Since the causes are not always

Zita's tips

* **Lose weight**. If you are obese, a weight reduction of 10 per cent of your body weight will boost your fertility (and regulate your cycle) as effectively as any assisted reproductive technique. Slow and gentle weight loss, with a gradual change in the types of food you eat, is a better method than crash dieting and calorie counting.

* **Women with PCOS** often have higher glucose levels and so are prone to diabetes. Losing excess

body fat will increase your insulin secretion, levelling out your blood sugar and reducing excess androgens. You may be prescribed drugs to help with this.

* **Weight loss** is particularly difficult if you have PCOS. Try not to be too discouraged or depressed, even if it is a long haul.

* **Balancing blood-sugar levels** is also very important for this condition. Choose foods that have a low glycaemic index, that

is "slow-releasing" or complex carbohydrates (see page 57 for examples), and introduce protein into each meal (see page 55).

* **Stress management** is vitally important if you suffer from PCOS since the adrenal glands react to stressful situations by releasing more testosterone, which further upsets hormonal balance.

* **Exercise regularly**: go for a brisk, 30-minute walk at least three times a week.

obvious, conventional drugs aim to reduce the symptoms of PCOS by:

* reducing the chances of cancerous changes in the endometrium (by prescribing the contraceptive pill or progesterone)
* improving fertility problems by inducing ovulation (anti-oestrogen drugs such as Clomid)
* reducing the masculinizing effects of the androgens (anti-androgen hormones or oestrogen).

Women are advised to lose weight if necessary, although this can be difficult for women with PCOS since weight gain is symptomatic of the condition. Insulin-sensitizing medication such as metformin may be prescribed as part of a calorie-controlled diet, but this anti-diabetic drug may have side effects (in 20 per cent of women) such as nausea, diarrhoea, abdominal discomfort or cramping.

Can complementary therapies help? If the condition is severe, natural remedies must only be used in a supportive capacity, accompanying conventional drugs prescribed to redress hormone imbalance. Treatments and remedies might include:

* acupuncture (see box, opposite)
* herbal medicines, which should always be prescribed by a qualified practitioner
* constitutional homeopathic remedies, which should also be prescribed by a qualified practitioner and preferably one with experience of treating fertility problems.

Case history

Elaine was diagnosed with PCOS in her early 20s. She conceived her two sons after a short course of Clomid, but when she tried for a third child, at the age of 34, she suffered unpleasant side effects from the drug, "feeling lousy with awful skin and horrible bloating". Ovulation tests did not look promising, so after six months Elaine came off Clomid and tried the progesterone supplement Provera instead. Again, there were unpleasant side effects, including manic mood swings, an erratic cycle with constant spotting and a feeling of being drained of energy. By this point **she had given up all hopes for a third child and simply wanted her erratic cycle to be sorted out.** Her doctor recommended the contraceptive pill, but Elaine wanted to try a more natural route. She decided to try acupuncture. Her first treatment eased the spotting and the second cleared it completely. Elaine continued to have weekly appointments and a month later she had a "normal" period. Concurrently, at Zita's suggestion, **Elaine visited a nutritionist who put her on vitamin and mineral supplements to redress various nutritional deficiencies.** She cut out red meat and made sure she drank a minimum of two litres of water a day. Acupuncture at this stage was geared solely at regulating her cycle, not starting ovulation, but her next period failed to appear. A pregnancy test was negative and there were no symptoms of pregnancy. A second test proved positive, however, and to her enormous surprise and delight, Elaine now has a daughter.

Diet and nutrition

Certain nutritional deficiencies are thought to be linked to miscarriage. If you are at risk, ensure you include certain key vitamins and minerals in your diet or take supplements.

* **Low levels of magnesium** are believed to be a factor. Oxidation, a process that damages cell membranes, can result in a loss of magnesium. Include magnesium-rich foods in your diet or take a supplement (see pages 61 and 63).

* **The antioxidant mineral selenium** protects cell membranes, helping to maintain magnesium levels. Women who miscarry have been found to have lower levels of selenium than women who go to term. Make sure you increase your dietary sources of this mineral (see page 63) or take a supplement.

* **Research suggests that levels of co-enzyme Q10** (see page 63) are lower in women who have miscarried. Production of co-Q10 in the body also depends on folic acid, vitamin B12 and betaine.

* **Vitamins A and E and beta-carotene levels tend to be** lower in women who have miscarried. Take a prenatal multivitamin supplement to raise your levels (see pages 59 and 61).

* **Vitamins B6 and B12 and folate** (see pages 60–61) are also essential. Deficiencies have been linked to miscarriage.

Recurrent miscarriage

Although losing a pregnancy is not the same as an inability to conceive, the impact of either can be devastating, both physically and emotionally. Too often couples are advised to "just keep trying", especially if they have already had a successful pregnancy. They won't be sent for tests until they have lost at least three pregnancies. New studies of immunology show, however, that if a miscarriage is the result of an auto-immune problem, subsequent pregnancies only serve to make the condition worse. If you are over 35, I suggest that you ask your doctor for tests after just one miscarriage.

Roughly half of all the eggs fertilized never progress to a viable pregnancy. Most women never know that they were pregnant, let alone that they have miscarried. More than 25 per cent lose a baby during the first trimester, and about one in 200 couples have two or more consecutive miscarriages.

What is it? Miscarriage is the loss of a pregnancy during the first 24 weeks of gestation. The loss of a pregnancy after 24 weeks is termed a stillbirth.

What causes it?
* The commonest cause of a miscarriage is a chromosomal abnormality of that pregnancy – in at least half of cases.
* Abnormal female anatomy, such as distortion of the uterine cavity or adhesions (scar tissue) caused by surgery or infection, is responsible for up to 10 per cent of miscarriages.
* Luteal phase defects (LPDs), such as inadequate progesterone production, are responsible for about a fifth of miscarriages.
* In as many as 15 per cent of cases of miscarriage the cause is unknown.
* Other possible causes include certain immune-system factors, endocrine (hormonal) disorders – such as poorly controlled diabetes or an under-active thyroid – defective sperm, infections of the reproductive tract or a problem with the time of implantation of an embryo.

Who is at risk? Women most at risk include those who:
* have had a miscarriage before
* are over the age of 35
* have anorexia
* are smokers
* have more than two alcoholic drinks a day
* drink coffee. Caffeine stays in the body of a pregnant woman much longer than in that of a non-pregnant woman. One study of 3,135 pregnant women showed that moderate to heavy coffee drinkers were more likely to have a late-first- or second-trimester miscarriage than non-coffee drinkers
* are exposed to X-rays or who spend long periods in planes

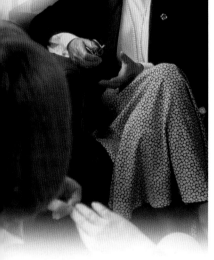

Counselling
or therapy can
help you come
to terms with
your loss.

* are excessively exposed to
environmental toxins such as
lead, mercury or organic solvents
* handle cytotoxic agents or
whose partners do
* have a serious illness
* use cocaine.
Other risk factors include:
* eating fish contaminated
with pollutants
* using laxatives, such as senna,
that stimulate smooth muscles,
including the uterus
* drinking chlorinated water
containing CBPs (chlorination
by-products). These are formed
when chlorine reacts with
organic material in the water.

How is it diagnosed? Medical
advances mean that 80 per cent
of the causes of miscarriage can

be identified and most problems
can be corrected or overcome.
The order of testing is usually:
* structural abnormalities
* problems with the luteal phase
* immune abnormalities (see also
pages 124–25)
* genetic diseases.

How is it treated conventionally?
There have been huge advances
in the field but there is also huge
controversy surrounding certain
forms of treatment.

Antibodies that might cause the
auto-immune disorder systemic
lupus erythematosus (SLE) – which
is inflammation of the body's
connective tissue causing damage
to internal organs – can be treated
with the drug prednisone.

Raised levels of natural killer
(NK) cells may be treated with an
immunoglobulin G (IgG) infusion
– a preparation of human-derived
antibodies – to prevent rejection
of an embryo.

Most structural defects can be
corrected surgically. In the case of
luteal phase defects, progesterone
may be prescribed during the
first 12 weeks of a pregnancy.
This hormone is responsible for
maintaining the endometrium,
which sustains the embryo/foetus
until the placenta has developed.

If there is a problem with
blocking antibodies, the mother
may be immunized with
concentrates of the father's white
blood cells, but this is a highly
controversial form of treatment
and is not widely available. Women

with abnormal blood-clotting often
carry the genes for a tendency to
encourage blood clotting. Clotting
problems may be treated with
low-dose aspirin, but some clinics
use heparin injections to thin the
blood, starting before pregnancy
occurs and continuing until 4–6
weeks after the birth. This is,
however, another controversial
form of treatment.

**Can complementary therapies
help?** As well as physical
treatment, you also have to deal
with the emotional devastation
of miscarriage. Feelings of guilt,
depression, failure, separation, loss,
envy and rage are all common.
Losing a baby can be especially
traumatic if you have had fertility
problems or you've miscarried
before. You need to work through
your feelings at your own pace
and with the right support (therapy,
counselling or a support group),
and learn how to deal with the
accompanying stress and anxiety.

Zita's tips

* **Seek advice** from a specialist
miscarriage clinic.

* **Talk things through** and
explore all the treatment
avenues very carefully.

* **Acupuncture** may strengthen
the kidneys. In Chinese
medicine, weak kidneys
are linked to miscarriage.

Immune problems

Although age is the biggest factor, about 40 per cent of "unexplained" infertility and 80 per cent of "unexplained" pregnancy loss (miscarriages that aren't the result of chromosomal defects, hormonal imbalance or abnormalities of the uterus) may be immunological.

Researching the problems

The medical world's understanding of reproductive immunology has increased significantly over the last few years, and a great deal of work is currently being done in both the UK and the US. There is still much disagreement between experts, however, about the causes of immune problems, and treatment remains controversial.

The area is a complex one, and specialists often work in narrow fields of research, so that it's hard to assess the whole picture. There is a lot of information published on the internet, but inevitably some of it is contradictory and even alarmist. If you have been diagnosed with an immune problem, my advice is to examine the evidence very carefully as it relates to you, and seek out a second opinion or even more.

Immune problems are increasingly believed to be a factor as far as some fertility problems are concerned, and may be the cause in cases of unexplained infertility. Antiphospholipid antibodies (APAs) are the most common example of abnormal immune reactions (see below).

What causes immune problems? The body naturally produces antibodies to fight off invasive and potentially harmful organisms. An embryo consists of tissue and genetic material from both you and your partner, and they combine to create a genetic structure and tissue type that is different from your own. The body's normal reaction is to reject "foreign" tissue, but during pregnancy your body should respond differently, forming a sort of protective blanket around the developing baby.

Some women's bodies are unable to do this, however. Their immune system behaves abnormally, either producing an auto-immune response, rejecting and attacking the developing embryonic cells as if they were an invading illness, or producing an allo-immune response, rejecting the father's genetic contribution (although this may not necessarily happen with a different partner). What this means is that the body does one of the following:

* Produces antiphospholipid antibodies (APAs). These attack the cells that build the placenta and its blood supply. This may cause problems initially with implantation, affect blood circulation between mother and embryo and increase the risk of miscarriage, intra-uterine growth retardation and pre-eclampsia.

* Produces anti-nuclear antibodies (ANAs). These attack the nuclei of cells in the uterus and placenta, causing inflammation and putting an embryo at risk. This may particularly affect women who suffer from conditions such as rheumatoid arthritis or systemic lupus erythematosus (SLE).

* Fails to produce blocking antibodies. Maternal blocking antibodies stop the immune system from attacking the foetus. Without them, the fertilized egg will be rejected and fail to implant. Sometimes the signal to switch on the maternal blocking antibodies is never triggered, perhaps because both parents have very similar genetic and tissue make-up.

✱ Produces an over-abundance of natural killer (NK) cells. These aggressively attack any rapidly growing or dividing cell in order to protect you from life-threatening diseases such as cancer. Unfortunately, however, they may be toxic as far as a developing foetus is concerned.

How are immune problems diagnosed?
Not everyone who has difficulty getting pregnant or whose IVF fails will have immune issues. However, if you have a history of any immune disease in the family, thyroid problems, two or more IVF failures with good embryos, or suffered recurrent miscarriages, you may have immune issues.

Blood tests are taken at six-week intervals to assess your immune status.

How are they treated conventionally?
Anticoagulants help to counteract clotting caused by APAs, so you may be prescribed low-dose aspirin to be taken daily or a combination of aspirin and injections of low-dose heparin (an anticoagulant derived from animal tissue). Treatment may be most effective if it is started before you conceive and then continued during the pregnancy.

Anti-nuclear antibodies can be treated with prednisone, a corticosteroid drug administered orally twice a day. This medication suppresses the inflammatory process and stabilizes the cell.

Recent studies have shown that intravenous infusions of intralipid, a soya-oil-based substance, may have a stabilizing effect on cell membranes making it harder for natural killer (NK) cells to attack. However, this treatment is not yet in widespread use, and isn't suitable for women with egg or soya allergies.

Case history

Andria, aged 35, started trying to conceive four years ago. She fell pregnant after nine months but miscarried at six weeks. Her doctor advised her to "keep trying". Ten months later she conceived, but miscarried at seven weeks; a third pregnancy ended at eight weeks. Still her doctor did not recommend investigations. Andria's husband is American, so she had tests in the US. No obvious cause of the miscarriages was identified. Immune therapy was discussed but dismissed as too controversial.

Back in the UK, **Andria was impatient to conceive so embarked on IVF. The first cycle was successful but she lost the baby at seven** weeks. She wanted to keep trying and begin another IVF cycle but her FSH (follicle-stimulating hormone) levels were consistently too high.

Meanwhile, research on the internet led her to fertility experts in Chicago and London. **She was found to be positive for antibodies and was therefore a good candidate for immune therapy.** While waiting for her FSH levels to come down, Andria had acupuncture. Following a holiday, she discovered she had conceived naturally. At five weeks, the optimum time for treatment, she was injected with her husband's white blood cells and began daily low-dose injections of a blood thinner. **At the time of writing, Andria is eight months pregnant.**

Hormonal imbalances

All aspects of a woman's reproductive life are influenced by the relative levels of the different female sex hormones in her body. Imbalances between them are responsible for a number of disorders.

Diet and nutrition

In most cases of hormonal and menstrual irregularities, dietary changes can improve the condition.

* **Eliminate all dairy products** from your diet.

* **Cut down** as much as possible on animal fats, processed foods and refined sugar.

* **Cut out coffee** – even if you're only on one cup a day – and any other drinks or food products containing caffeine.

* **Increase the amount of fibre** in your diet to help eliminate excess oestrogen (unless you already consume a lot of fibre) and eat more foods containing phyto-oestrogens (see page 31).

* **Avoid alcohol** altogether if you can, or limit yourself to an occasional drink.

* **Take a good multivitamin** and mineral supplement daily. Make sure you have sufficient intakes of calcium, magnesium and vitamin B6 in particular (see pages 59–64).

* **Ensure that your diet contains** enough essential fatty acids (see pages 63–64); sources include oily fish, nuts and seeds, evening primrose oil, linseed oil, sesame oil, walnut oil and sunflower oil.

Cycle problems

There is no direct link between certain menstrual irregularities and fertility problems (with the exception of luteal phase defects), but it follows that underlying hormonal, nutritional or emotional imbalances that contribute to cycle problems may also be a factor in reduced fertility. Until a balance has been restored, it may be difficult to conceive. The nature of hormonal imbalance varies but it is closely linked to nutritional deficiencies and high intakes of processed foods, fats and caffeine. A good diet is an essential part of any treatment plan (see box, left).

PMS

Between 25 and 100 per cent of women are believed to suffer from premenstrual syndrome and 10 per cent are seriously debilitated. It is more common in women aged 35–45, but certain symptoms may be signs of perimenopause.

PMS includes a range of symptoms that recur cyclically, usually between 12 and 5 days before menstruation. They disappear once a period starts. Symptoms are the result of a complex interaction of emotional, physical and genetic factors, but are generally related to oestrogen and progesterone imbalances. Depending on the type of PMS you have, symptoms may include headaches, cravings, fatigue, dizziness and fainting, abdominal bloating and cramping, breast tenderness, back pain, mood swings, insomnia, irritability, tearfulness, social withdrawal, depression and forgetfulness.

PMS is often triggered by hormonal changes, for example if a woman stops taking the pill, if she is approaching menopause or if she has had a serious emotional trauma. Women may also be at risk if they have a diet high in processed foods, refined sugar, dairy products and animal fat but low in whole grains, fruit and vegetables; they have low levels of magnesium, selenium and vitamins B-complex, C and E; they are overweight; they don't exercise enough; or they suffer chronic stress leading to adrenal exhaustion and oestrogen dominance.

Conventional drugs such as painkillers, antidepressants, diuretics or synthetic progesterone may relieve symptoms, but they do not tackle the underlying cause and

Many women find PMS symptoms are worse during autumn and winter.

may have unpleasant side effects. Rather than addressing specific symptoms, complementary medicine views PMS as a wake-up call to alert you to underlying imbalances. Acupuncture or constitutional homeopathy may help tackle the underlying causes of hormonal imbalance. Herbal remedies such as chaste-tree berry may relieve symptoms, but should only be taken under supervision.

Menorrhagia

This describes excessive menstrual bleeding that may be the result of an oestrogen or progesterone imbalance. Periods are regular but blood flow is extremely heavy and may be long-lasting and contain large clots. Menorrhagia can lead to anaemia and chronic fatigue. It is most common in women in their 40s, and may be related to endometriosis (see pages 114–16), ovarian cysts (see pages 119–21), pelvic inflammatory disease (PID, see page 108), thyroid problems (see pages 106–107) or fibroids (see pages 117–19).

Conventional treatment varies, depending on the cause, but may take the form of prostaglandin inhibitors (such as ibuprofen) or synthetic progesterone. A number of self-help measures may help to improve this condition, including regular exercise and stress relief, as well as good nutrition (see box, opposite). Herbal medicine may be useful to help regulate bleeding or clear oestrogen. Homeopathy or acupuncture may also help.

Dysmenorrhoea

This describes severe pain and cramping during menstruation, felt in the lower back, abdomen and inner thighs. It is thought to be related to an oestrogen and progesterone imbalance. If it is related to endometriosis or other pelvic disease it is felt more as a dull ache in the lower back and pelvic area (and is known as secondary dysmenorrhoea). Up to 60 per cent of women suffer from menstrual cramps, some of them being severely debilitated.

Zita's tips

* **Allow yourself time for self-nurturing** – to be alone to rest quietly, reflect and switch off from daily stresses and strains. The reduction of stress is important for the relief of many cycle problems, preventing adrenal exhaustion and the resulting oestrogen dominance.

* **Do at least 20 minutes' aerobic exercise** at least three times a week to help relieve stress, improve general circulation and release endorphins.

* **Eat small meals at regular intervals** so that blood-sugar levels do not fall too low.

* **Try to get at least two hours of bright light** or sunshine every day.

* **Try homeopathic remedies** to relieve your particular symptoms, especially those of PMS; take every 12 hours for 3 days before the onset of symptoms:
Sepia 30c if you are irritable, tearful, emotionally flat or craving sweet or salty foods.

Pulsatilla 30c if you are tearful or nauseous and you have painful breasts and irregular periods.
Natrum mur 30c if you are low and irritable and have water retention and swollen breasts.
Calcarea 30c if you are tired, lethargic and clumsy and your breasts are swollen and painful.
Lycopodium 30c if you are bad-tempered and crave sweet things.
Causticum 30c if you are pessimistic and over-sensitive, with urinary problems and colicky pains.

Conventional treatment takes the form of anti-inflammatory drugs or the contraceptive pill, which is obviously not a good idea if you are trying to get pregnant. Gentle exercise prior to a period, stress-reduction techniques and good nutrition (see box on page 126) are useful self-help measures.

Amenorrhoea

As with other menstrual problems, amenorrhoea is an indication of hormonal and nutritional imbalance. Periods stop for several months, not because of pregnancy or menopause but as a result of temporary failure of the ovaries and the pituitary gland.

The condition is sometimes accompanied by an under-active thyroid (see pages 106–07), and may be a symptom of polycystic ovary syndrome (see PCOS, pages 119–21). You may also be at risk if you suffer great weight loss, take intense physical exercise, come off the pill, have extreme emotional stress, are obese, take certain drugs that increase prolactin levels or if you have nutritional deficiencies.

Diet is the best place to start with this problem, especially maintaining a good balance of carbohydrates, fat and protein, eating plenty of whole grains and pulses and taking a multivitamin and mineral supplement (see also box on page 126). Oestrogen replacement therapy is the conventional treatment.

Luteal phase defect (LPD)

This is technically an ovulation disorder resulting from hormonal imbalance and causing conception difficulties. If the luteal phase (see pages 10–11) is shorter than normal, insufficient progesterone is available to maintain a fertilized egg until it implants. Progesterone deficiency may be associated with the faulty secretion of luteinizing hormone (LH) and hence failed ovulation. Drug treatment may include ovulation stimulation or progesterone supplementation.

Predicting ovulation

Women who have **irregular menstrual cycles** may find it hard to predict when they ovulate. Many use **ovulation kits** which identify the LH surge (see page 10). Women with long or short cycles may need **follicular tracking**. This is the use of **ultrasound scanning** at weekly intervals during a woman's cycle to determine when ovulation has taken place. The advantage of this is that a woman doesn't have to take medication to regulate her cycle.

Zita's tips

There are several self-help measures that may encourage your FSH levels to come down.

* **Take regular, gentle exercise** but nothing too strenuous.

* **Try to lose excess weight** if you are overweight.

* **Practise** meditation and deep-breathing techniques on a regular basis in order to reduce stress and improve relaxation.

Raised FSH levels

Levels of follicle-stimulating hormone (FSH) tend to fluctuate during a woman's monthly cycle throughout her 30s and early 40s as perimenopause approaches (see page 16–17). Few women have any idea about their FSH levels, however, until they start trying for a baby. I see many women who wait from month to month for their FSH levels to come down, having discovered that they have problems conceiving and while they wait to start IVF (in vitro fertilization) treatment.

What is it? FSH is a hormone released by the pituitary gland to encourage an egg to ripen and mature (see pages 10–11). FSH levels give a good indication of ovarian reserve (see page 16). If levels are raised, as your body tries to stimulate ovulation, it is likely that egg quality will be poor.

What causes it? FSH levels do fluctuate naturally, especially in reaction to stress, but raised levels may indicate that perimenopause or menopause is imminent or has already started. This condition may also indicate that ovulation has not occurred. Some women do, however, go on to have a successful pregnancy, although this is uncommon. Egg quality tends to decline significantly for some women in their 30s and at an even faster rate during their early 40s. By the age of 45, the chances of getting pregnant are greatly decreased, as older women have older eggs which may carry chromosome abnormalities. They are also more likely to miscarry. However, egg quality in a particular individual may be average for her age, better than average or worse than average.

What are the symptoms? There are no symptoms of raised FSH levels, and very often the first thing a women knows about the significance of her FSH levels is following the results of a routine blood test that she might have as part of fertility testing procedures (see page 99) if she finds she is having difficulty conceiving.

How is it diagnosed? A routine blood test is done on days 2–4 of the menstrual cycle (or, if a period has been missed, at any time). This test is used to diagnose or evaluate disorders of the pituitary gland or reproductive system.

How is it treated conventionally? There is currently no conventional treatment for raised FSH levels.

Can complementary therapies help? I use acupuncture to help lower raised FSH levels with some degree of success, but it does depend on how high the levels are to start with. I treat a number of important acupoints for hormone regulation and reproduction.

There are a number of general lifestyle factors to be considered (see Zita's Tips, opposite), and diet is important (see box, right).

Spend time relaxing, using deep-breathing techniques and meditating on the colour blue.

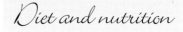

Diet and nutrition

There are a number of dietary measures you can put into effect to try to bring down your FSH levels.

* **Put yourself on a detoxifying programme,** including drinking at least 2 litres (3.5 pints) of still bottled or filtered water a day, cutting down your salt intake and avoiding coffee, tea and sugary and carbonated drinks. Drink hot water and lemon juice instead. (See also pages 50–53.)

* **Consult a qualified herbalist** about taking a daily supplement of chaste-tree berry (*Vitex agnus castus*), which may help to lower elevated FSH levels.

* **Take a B-complex supplement,** containing 50mg of B6, and a zinc supplement to help regulate hormones generally.

* **Take 1000mg of essential fatty acids a day,** either evening primrose oil or fish oils.

* **Eat pulses, onions and garlic** to help the liver to break down oestrogen, and cabbage to increase the rate at which the liver converts oestrogen into its water-soluble form so that it can be excreted from the body.

* **Eat foods containing phyto-oestrogens** – such as pulses, linseeds, alfalfa sprouts, oats, cabbage and sprouts – which bind to oestrogen receptors, causing a weak oestrogen-like response (see also page 31). This will help to balance hormones.

Raised prolactin levels

Prolactin levels are usually high during pregnancy and lactation (see also page 100). Abnormally high prolactin levels may upset hormonal balance and interfere with normal ovulation and the luteal phase following the release of an egg (see pages 10–11). This is the reason why nursing mothers rarely become pregnant. Once prolactin levels are normalized, ovulation resumes in most cases.

What is it? Prolactin is a hormone that is produced by the pituitary gland, principally to prepare the breasts for producing milk after childbirth. Levels are normally low in non-pregnant women. The release of prolactin is suppressed by dopamine, a neurotransmitter produced in the brain. Any reduction in the production of dopamine not only allows prolactin levels to rise but

also interferes with the production of gonadotrophin-releasing hormone (GnRH). This in turn affects the manufacture of follicle-stimulating hormone (FHS) and luteinizing hormone (LH). The result of this hormonal imbalance is menstrual dysfunction (irregular periods) and disrupted ovulation.

What causes it? High levels of prolactin, or hyperprolactinaemia, can be caused by or associated with:
* certain drugs, including blood pressure medication, antidepressants and anaesthetics
* prolonged periods of stress
* excessive amounts of exercise
* an under-active thyroid (see pages 106–07)
* polycystic ovary syndrome (PCOS) – see pages 119–21
* small, non-cancerous tumours (prolactinomas) in the pituitary gland that either cause more prolactin to be secreted or prevent dopamine from reaching prolactin-producing cells.

What are the symptoms? These include menstrual irregularities, such as absent periods, and ovulatory dysfunction, the inappropriate production of breast milk and a loss of libido.

Who is at risk? Anyone suffering from high levels of stress, hypothyroidism or anorexia or taking certain drugs (see above) is at risk of raised prolactin levels.

Zita's tips

There are several self-help and lifestyle measures that may help lower raised prolactin levels.

* **Use relaxation** and stress-management techniques to reduce the impact of stress.

* **Avoid strenuous exercise** for prolonged periods.

* **Avoid alcohol,** especially beer.

Diet and nutrition

Dietary measures recommended for lowering raised prolactin levels include **increased amounts of zinc and vitamin B6,** both of which are necessary for the normal synthesis of dopamine. **Good food sources** of zinc include lean meats, fish and seafood, chicken, eggs, pumpkin and sunflower seeds, rye, oats and whole grains, while for **B6, which aids the absorption of zinc,** they are green leafy vegetables, whole grains, molasses, nuts, brown rice, egg yolks, organ meats, fish, poultry, pulses and seeds.

How is it diagnosed? A blood test will measure prolactin levels.

How is it treated conventionally? Levels can be brought down with the drugs bromocriptine (brand name Parlodel), a synthetic form of dopamine, or cabergoline (brand name Dostinex). If a tumour is responsible for raised levels, it can often be treated successfully with drugs and will only occasionally require surgery.

Can complementary therapies help? The herb chaste-tree berry (*Vitex agnus castus*) has been shown to mimic the action of dopamine and may help to lower prolactin levels after use for about three months. Make sure you consult a qualified practitioner. Acupuncture may help to balance hormone levels.

Herbs for hormonal imbalance

Some herbs act as hormonal regulators, while others are good uterine tonics. You should never self-subscribe herbal remedies – always seek the supervision of a qualified herbalist, and stop taking any remedies once you become pregnant.

A number of herbal remedies might be recommended by a practitioner. These include:

* **Chaste-tree berry** (*Vitex agnus castus*), a hormonal regulator that stimulates the release of luteinizing hormone (LH) and prolactin, decreases the secretion of follicle-stimulating hormone (FSH) and promotes ovulation. This herb is the most extensively researched in connection with the treatment of hormonal problems in women. It is particularly useful for luteal phase defects (see page 128), anovulation (no ovulation) and polymenorrhoea (very frequent periods). Do not use chaste-tree berry if you might be pregnant or if you have polycystic ovaries.

* **Siberian ginseng** (*Eleutherococcus senticosus*), which may help to regulate hormones and promote general health and vitality. It supports the adrenal glands and helps to reduce stress levels.

* **Dong quai** (*Angelica sinensis*), which can tone a weak uterus and regulate hormones and the menstrual cycle. This should be taken under supervision since too much can cause heavy periods.

* **Red clover** (*Trifolium pratense*), which contains oestrogen-like compounds.

* **Liquorice** (*Glycyrrhiza spp.*), which can help women who have irregular periods and those who have elevated testosterone and low levels of oestrogen. This herb has a high sodium content and intakes must be supervised.

* **Black cohosh** (*Cimicifuga racemosa*), which stimulates the release of LH and contains isoflavone constituents that have oestrogen-like activity, that is they bind to oestrogen receptors. Do not confuse with blue cohosh.

* **Mexican wild yam** (*Dioscorea villosa*), which contains components of progesterone and encourages the release of this hormone after ovulation.

* **Red raspberry leaf** (*Rubus idaeus*) is a uterine tonic and hormone regulator. Take this preconceptually but not during the first six months of pregnancy.

Red clover blossom contains oestrogen-like compounds.

* **Motherwort** (*Leonurus spp.*), a uterine tonic that tones the female reproductive system.

* **Squaw vine** (*Mitchella repens*), a uterine tonic that provides a calcium- and iron-rich remedy for hormonal imbalance and irregular periods.

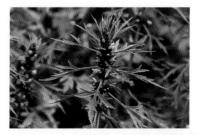

Motherwort tones the uterus and the female reproductive system.

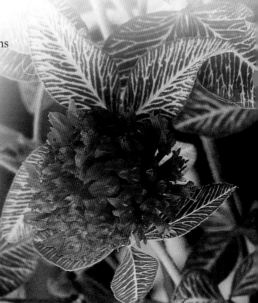

Male fertility tests

In as many as half the couples who are unable to conceive, it is the man who has a fertility problem. It is important, therefore, that your partner is involved in the diagnostic process. Many conditions affecting male fertility (see pages 138–41) are symptomless, so skilled investigation is necessary in order to identify them.

Check sperm first

I always suggest to couples that a sperm check is one of the first tests to have; it's relatively quick and straightforward. Men are often reluctant to take action before a specific problem has been found and to take a test that may identify them as the one with the problem. Your partner will have to be prepared to give a detailed personal and medical history to your doctor or a consultant, including his previous sexual activity. Coping with a negative result and finding somebody to talk to about it, other than you, isn't easy, even though the problem is far more common than most people, especially men, imagine. You will need to be prepared to handle all these issues sensitively.

Just as for women, there are many different factors and combinations of factors that give rise to fertility problems in men. The sequence of tests for a man is as follows:

* **level one** physical examination and analysis of a semen sample
* **level two** hormone assessment
* **level three** further tests including physical examination, scanning, biopsy and genetic tests.

The first thing your doctor or fertility consultant will do is take details about your partner's medical and sexual history.

Level one: physical examination & semen analysis

Looking for the obvious

On your partner's first visit to the doctor, your doctor will check the testicles visually and manually for varicocele (see page 139), undescended testicles or any other visible evidence of physiological problems (see pages 140–41).

Analysing semen

Semen assessment is a simple and convenient way of measuring a man's potential fertility. There are many different reasons why he might have abnormal sperm – semen analysis may well pinpoint the cause (see pages 138–41).

One common misconception about semen quality is that male fertility is linked to virility. If a man receives a poor semen assessment, he may feel crushed on two counts – the implications for his prospects of becoming a father, and his perceived reflection on his status as a man. Many men are reluctant to admit the problem to their peers, and make other excuses for having to give up alcohol, for example, in order to improve their sperm count.

Providing a sample

At a fertility clinic, your partner will be asked to ejaculate into a sterile container. The sample is examined under a microscope. It sounds simple, but masturbating to order is not always easy, especially in that environment. It can be easily perceived as an embarrassing, uncomfortable and humiliating experience, the ultimate invasion of privacy.

If your partner has difficulty producing a sample for whatever reason, or your religion forbids masturbation, it is possible to use non-spermicidal, non-latex condoms at home. He will need to get the sample to the clinic within an hour for immediate assessment, however. Also, semen needs to be transported at body temperature, since cold kills sperm. Your clinic will advise you how to do this. Consider asking them to freeze and bank a supply of semen in case your partner is unable to produce a sample at a critical point in a procedure. If his difficulty is the result of impotency caused by a physiological or a psychological problem (if he was abused as a child, for example), specialist counselling may help.

Your partner should refrain from ejaculation for 2–4 days before providing a sample. In specific cases, he may be asked to give a urine sample immediately after ejaculation – this will be used to check for retrograde ejaculation (see page 141). Bear in mind that sperm can take up to 100 days to mature (see pages 14–15), so it is worth mentioning any illnesses he's had in the last three months that may have affected the condition of the sperm, any medication he has taken or is taking, excessive heat he has experienced (for example, in a sauna) and excess weight he is carrying. Clearly it might be dangerous to stop taking certain prescribed drugs. The fact is that doctors do not know the cause of some sperm problems, but discuss all medication with the consultant.

The results of semen analysis are usually available quickly, so make an early follow-up appointment to discuss them

Specialist analysis

It is essential that the semen assessment is done properly, in a fertility clinic or **specialist andrology lab.** Many National Health Service (NHS) hospitals also offer this service. It is also vitally important that the results are **properly interpreted** — not all doctors or even gynaecologists have the necessary specialist experience. Valuable time can be wasted if a couple is told their sperm is fine but a faulty test or misinterpretation has failed to reveal a problem.

Go to your local fertility clinic or, if necessary, pay for a **private assessment** (some private health insurance policies may cover this) – it is not hugely expensive and is definitely **money well spent.**

with your doctor. Sperm quality is easily affected by variables such as health and stress, so your partner may have to give further samples over the next few months, even if the first test is normal or borderline. Do not be in too much of a hurry to retest. Allow time for lifestyle or dietary improvements to take effect.

Understanding the results

There are several different aspects of semen analysis, each with its parameters with regard to what is considered "normal" fertility.

Appearance Normal semen is opalescent and greyish. Yellow semen might indicate high intakes of vitamin supplements, which is not a problem; high levels of flavoproteins resulting from long abstinence, which is easily remedied; or, rarely, jaundice. A reddish colour may mean there are red blood cells in the semen. This may indicate an infection so further investigation will be necessary (see page 137).

Volume The average ejaculate contains about 2ml, less than half a teaspoon. Many men are surprised and apologetic about this. A high volume means a diluted concentration of sperm. Less than 1ml may indicate a pathological problem, such as a current or past infection (for example, a sexually transmitted infection, or STI) which has blocked the ejaculatory ducts

producing seminal fluid. Low volume may mean retrograde ejaculation or problems with accessory glands, seminal vesicles or the prostate. Low volume as well as no sperm might indicate a condition such as congenital bi-lateral absence of the vas deferens (CBAVD – see page 141). Your partner might then be referred to a urologist to treat the problem or referred for an assisted reproductive technique (ART – see page 144).

Viscosity and liquefaction
Normal ejaculate is initially very viscous but becomes runny after about 10 minutes due to the action of enzymes. If this does not occur within about an hour, sperm find it difficult to swim up the cervix. This is not a serious problem – sperm can be washed and re-suspended in a special solution before being injected into the uterus.

Acidity Semen is normally quite alkaline (with a pH rarely below 7; the norm is between 7.2 and 8.0). Ejaculate that is acidic and without sperm is probably the result of CBAVD (see above).

Agglutination This means that motile sperm stick to one other. It usually indicates the presence of anti-sperm antibodies (see page 140 and right) – proteins that coat sperm and bind to cervical mucus, preventing sperm from moving towards an egg or fertilizing it.

This is a common cause of failed IVF. Some antibodies are cytotoxic, which means they destroy sperm. A MAR (mixed agglutination reaction) test (see below) will be necessary if sperm are sticking.

Antibodies Antibodies are not usually present in semen. They are caused by injury or surgery, such as vasectomy reversal or hernia repair, when a breakdown in the blood-testes barrier allows blood and testicular tissue to come into contact. Anti-sperm antibodies may be present in semen even if there is no agglutination (see above). It is only when they are present on sperm at relatively high levels that fertility may be affected. As well as preventing sperm from moving, antibodies may coat the sperm heads, making it difficult for them to recognize an egg and fertilize it.

Antibody tests are expensive and tend not to be done routinely until other factors have been eliminated. In vitro fertilization (see pages 154–81) with intra-cytoplasmic sperm injection (ICSI, see page 174) or intra-uterine insemination (IUI, see pages 152–53) may be suggested, depending on test results. Steroid treatment is another option.

MAR (mixed agglutination reaction) This test (also known as an immunobead test) is very important for antibodies but is often overlooked in standard NHS (National Health Service) semen analysis, and you may need to pay for it to be done at a fertility clinic. If it shows less than 50 per cent binding, antibody levels should not affect your partner's fertility.

Round cell concentration

Round cells are either immature sperm cells or white blood cells. A concentration of more than 1 million per 1ml white blood cells or 5 million round cells may indicate an infection. Prognosis depends on severity – a course of antibiotics may clear up the problem, but a serious infection can result in permanent damage.

Sperm concentration This is the number of sperm in semen. A count of at least 20 million per 1ml is considered to be normally fertile (the average is 60–80 million/ml). A lower count is termed oligozoospermia. No sperm in the semen is known as azoospermia. Frequent ejaculation reduces the concentration. Well-documented evidence shows that sperm count is hugely affected by lifestyle factors – intakes of caffeine, tobacco, alcohol and recreational drugs, diet, exercise and stress levels. Lifestyle changes can make a big difference and may be all a man needs to do to increase the count. Numbers of sperm may also be affected by a previous STI. A concentration of less than 5 million per 1ml

Semen assessment

Patient: John Smith	DOB: 3 February
Address: 2 Long Lane	Reference No: JS209W
Newtown	Referring Practitioner: Zita West
Tel: 3456789	Date: 6th April

Duration of abstinence (days): 3

Interval between ejaculation and start of analysis (mins): 20

	Sample	Normal range
Appearance	Normal	
Volume (ml)	3.2ml	2ml or more
Viscosity	Normal	
Liquefaction	Complete	Complete within 60 mins
pH	8.0	7.2 or more
Agglutination	Some	None
MAR Test for IgG (% with adherent particles)	4% binding Head 0 Tail 4 Midpiece 0	<10% absence of antibodies <50% may not affect fertility
MAR Test for IgA (% with adherent particles)	2% binding Head 0 Tail 2 Midpiece 0	<10% absence of antibodies <50% may not affect fertility
Round cell concentration (10^6/ml)	0.3	5 x 10^6/ml or less (<1 x 10^6/ml leukocytes)
Sperm concentration (10^6/ml)	47	20 x 10^6/ml or more
Total no. of sperm (10^6)	150	40 x 10^6 per ejaculate or more
Motility (% a + b + c)	62	50% or more (a + b) or 25% or more (a)
(a) rapid progression	42	
(b) slow progression	16	
(c) non-progressive motility	4	
(d) immotile	38	
Morphology (% abnormal forms)	92	multicentre studies now in progress
– **normal**	8	
– head defects	89	
– neck or midpiece defects	43	
– tail defects	12	
– cytoplasmic droplets	2	
Teratozoospermia index (TZI) (total no. defects/no. sperm with defects)	1.59	1.6 or less

Comments *High proportion of abnormal forms (Teratozoopermia) – multiple defects; most sperm have round or amorphous heads. All other parameters within normal reference range.*

Semen analysis The results your partner gets back may look something like this, although forms vary from clinic to clinic. Your consultant will explain the findings very carefully, but ask questions if you do not fully understand the implications.

Case history

Stephen, 35, had been trying to conceive a baby with his wife, Wendy, for more than a year. He wasn't expecting anything untoward from his sperm analysis and was devastated when the count was zero. Stephen became depressed as further testing revealed hormonal imbalance and testicular failure. His doctor was rather abrupt when outlining the couple's options – donor sperm or adoption. After counselling, Stephen and Wendy opted for donor insemination and now feel much more positive having made the decision.

indicates that your partner may have a genetic chromosomal defect, which might result, for example, in you miscarrying. If your partner has a Y-chromosome deletion, it affects the way sperm are made and cannot be corrected. An assisted reproductive technology (ART) with pre-implantation genetic diagnosis may be recommended. Donor insemination is also a possibility. If the count is very

low or zero, your partner will be referred to a urologist for blood tests (see Level 2, right) or a testicular biopsy.

Motility Sperm need to be good swimmers and move rapidly in straight lines. Motility describes the proportion of moving sperm and is affected both by lifestyle and frequency of ejaculation. After a long period of abstinence, semen will contain many dead and immotile sperm, so a man needs to have intercourse within three days of a sperm test – but not on the same morning or else the concentration will be lowered. Poor sperm motility is known as asthenozoospermia.

Progression describes the way in which the sperm are moving and is graded as follows:
* rapid progression in straight lines
* slow progression with erratic movement
* non-progressive motility – the sperm are twitching but not moving forwards
* immotile.

Normal, fertile sperm usually includes at least 50 per cent first and second progression categories, or 25 per cent first category. If a man's sperm are mainly third and fourth categories, he may have a serious fertility problem.

Many men mistakenly believe that the occasional alcoholic binge does not affect the quality of their sperm. In fact, just one

evening of heavy drinking will seriously damage sperm, and it could take three months for the sperm count to be restored.

Morphology This refers to the shape of sperm. Abnormalities include large or small heads, irregularly shaped heads, two heads or coiled tails. Poor morphology is known as teratozoospermia. According to the World Health Organization, 4 per cent or more normal sperm constitutes normal fertility. Levels below 4 per cent may indicate sub-fertility. Morphology is affected by lifestyle and occasionally genetic defects. Age is also significant: sperm quality deteriorates beyond 40 and the number of abnormal sperm increases over time. Men can, however, produce healthy sperm all their lives.

Assessing male fertility

Fertility (or sub-fertility) is a matter of degree. Sub-optimal parameters do not mean a man is infertile, but he might find it difficult to conceive naturally. It is almost impossible to predict whether or not a man can become a biological father; absolute sterility (the absence of sperm in either ejaculate or testes) is rare.

The next step will depend upon the results of semen analysis. If sperm count is low and does not improve after a few months of lifestyle changes, further testing will be recommended.

Level two: hormone assessment

This is not necessary very often. A simple blood test will indicate levels of the key sex hormones – FSH (follicle-stimulating hormone), LH (luteinizing hormone), prolactin and testosterone. LH stimulates the production of testosterone – necessary for the development of healthy sperm – in the testicles. Prolactin can interfere with LH-induced testosterone production. FSH is essential for sperm development. Results falling either side of the expected range indicate hormonal imbalance, which has a number of causes (see page 140). Treatment is by hormone-replacement drugs.

Understanding the results

The interpretation of hormone results is complex; the following examples are simplified. If your partner has high levels of FSH and LH and low testosterone levels, he may have testicular failure (see pages 140–41). A biopsy can determine whether or not it is possible to retrieve sperm for ICSI (intra-cytoplasmic sperm injection – see page 174), a procedure whereby sperm are injected into an egg. Another option would be the use of donor sperm (see page 182). Low levels of testosterone and FSH may indicate hypothalamic dysfunction (see page 140).

The hormonal control of sperm production may also be affected by underlying medical conditions, such as liver disease. If your partner's hormone levels appear normal, his consultant may recommend other, specifically targeted tests.

Level three: further tests

Further investigation may be recommended to determine whether or not there is damage to the testes, any other physiological damage or genetic defects.

Cell culture This can identify infection. Testicular inflammation may lead to reduced testosterone and therefore no sperm production. On the other hand, severe infection may cause a permanent obstruction, leading to azoospermia.

Ultrasound scanning This is used to examine the scrotum, testes, epididymis, prostate and seminal vesicles. It can detect infection and inflammation, the absence of the vas deferens (CBAVD), obstruction and tumours. Varicocele diagnosis uses Doppler ultrasonography. Surgery to unblock an obstruction may be helpful in some cases, but the benefits of surgery for solving fertility problems are still open to debate. Alternatively, sperm may be removed surgically from behind the obstruction and used in an assisted reproductive technique such as ICSI (see above).

Testicular biopsy This is used to determine whether or not there is any sperm development in the testicular tissue. This test is useful if all other tests are normal and yet there is an unexplained absence of sperm in the semen.

Chromosome testing Genetic evaluation may be offered to men who have sperm counts of fewer than 5 million per 1ml. About 4 per cent of men with such a low count, and up to 15 per cent of those with no sperm, have a chromosomal abnormality. Chromosome testing will also be offered to men with CBAVD because of its association with cystic fibrosis, which could be inherited by any offspring.

If your partner has severe oligozoospermia (see page 135), non-obstructive azoospermia (see page 141), or an absence of sperm due to a blockage, the cause may be a chromosome abnormality. Other genetic causes for male infertility include Young's syndrome, Kartagener's syndrome or Klinefelter's syndrome (see page 141). Potential genetic problems are investigated by means of blood tests. Depending on the results, you may be offered an assisted reproductive technique (see page 144) and genetic counselling.

Male fertility problems

Fertility has traditionally been considered the woman's "responsibility". In fact, female factors alone account for 35–40 per cent of fertility problems, male factors alone are the cause in 30–35 per cent of cases, and in the rest there is a combined problem. Sperm-quality problems can often be improved.

Sperm and fertility

In order to impregnate a woman naturally and successfully, a man must first produce sperm that are capable of finding their way to the egg and then they must be able to fertilize it. For this to be possible, sperm need to be produced in sufficient quantities, be of good enough quality and be fit enough to complete what amounts to a herculean task. If a man's production of healthy sperm is compromised in any way, it may affect a couple's fertility. In most cases, the reason for poor sperm quality is not known (idiopathic).

Declining sperm counts

Average sperm counts are in decline. They have decreased rapidly in the last 50 years (from 113 million per ml to around 70 million per ml). The percentage of sperm with abnormalities has increased 12-fold and sperm motility has decreased. As a practitioner, I've noticed increasingly over the last few years that greater numbers of men are coming to me with fertility problems. There are many theories about the cause of the decline – it is probably the result of a combination of factors.

The causes of male infertility

Generally, male infertility can be grouped into four major categories: abnormal sperm; defective hormone production; damage to the testes and other physiological problems – such as ejaculation problems; and genetic problems.

In at least 30 per cent of male infertility cases, the cause is never determined; in 3–5 per cent of cases, the cause is hormonal in origin; in at least 30 per cent, problems are thought to be due to the effects of varicocele; 10–20 per cent result from infections; 6–7 per cent of cases are due to sperm obstruction; and 6–7 per cent of problems are ultimately found to be of genetic origin.

It is important to support your partner if he finds he is unable to conceive.

Abnormal sperm

In some men with apparent fertility problems, their hormonal balance and testes appear fine, but the sperm they produce are abnormal. Sperm can be damaged in a number of ways. Some men have great-looking sperm – a high count, excellent motility and a good shape – yet the sperm are not able to fertilize an egg. There are so many events occurring at the molecular level that are required for normal fertilization to take place, that if there is a problem with any one of them, fertilization will be compromised. At this level, it is almost impossible to diagnose the cause, and in most cases the reason for infertility remains unexplained.

Immotile sperm Kartagener's syndrome, also known as immotile cilia syndrome, is a condition in which normal quantities of sperm are produced but their tails do not enable them to move. Even though they cannot move, as long as the sperm are alive and healthy in all other respects, they can be removed from a man and injected into a woman's eggs in order to fertilize them.

Environmental toxins We hear a lot about the impact of toxins on sperm (see pages 75–76). Some of them, including cigarette smoke, contain what are known as reactive oxygen species. These molecules are also produced by white blood cells in response to infection and by damaged sperm themselves. The oxidizing effects of reactive oxygen species are thought to be responsible for greater numbers of abnormal sperm. Taking an antioxidant supplement (see pages 59–63) may help to reduce the amounts of these molecules in semen.

Varicocele Varicocele is a condition that is similar to varicose veins in the testicular area. Some men with varicocele experience no fertility problems, while other men do. Varicocele is found to be quite common among infertile men. The condition results in poor blood flow and is generally believed to be responsible for sperm damage.

Your partner's feelings

Receiving a poor diagnosis, and particularly the discovery that he has a low or non-existent sperm count, can have a devastating effect on a man. He may feel inadequate and have low self-esteem. **If he receives a poor semen assessment, as well as thinking his virility has been undermined, he may blame himself for letting you down.** *These feelings will be accentuated if the quality of his sperm cannot be improved and as a couple you need fertility treatment to conceive. He will have to stand by while you undergo drug therapy and invasive procedures, while the worst he will have to endure, except in a few unusual cases, is to ejaculate repeatedly into a cup.* **He may be withdrawn or lose interest in sex; he may even become impotent.**

It is important that you keep talking to each other, although he may find it difficult under the circumstances. **Don't misinterpret his reactions as lack of concern.** *Remember that more than 40 per cent of all fertility problems occur in males; 2 per cent of men produce no sperm at all. There has been a marked decline in sperm quality, and male infertility is a growing problem.*

Antibodies In some cases, the inability of sperm to fertilize an egg may be due to antibodies in the semen. Anti-sperm antibodies only affect fertility, however, if they actually coat the sperm and occur in relatively high concentrations. This is known as immunological infertility. Surgery, such as for hernia repair, or vasectomy reversal, usually results in the presence of anti-sperm antibodies.

Defective hormone production

Men often associate hormones with women's reproductive cycles, little realizing that hormones have a huge impact on their own fertility (see pages 14–15). Specific hormonal imbalance can affect a man's fertility. Follicle-stimulating hormone (FSH) and luteinizing hormone (LH), the gonadotrophin hormones, are released from the pituitary gland to stimulate testosterone production. A lack of these hormones means a lack of testosterone and impaired sperm production. This is known as hypogonadotropic hypogonadism. It may be the result of a genetic defect, such as Kallmann syndrome, or damage to the pituitary gland or hypothalamus as a result of another medical condition, such as a brain tumour. It may even be caused by malnutrition or fasting.

General hormonal imbalance may be caused by certain medical conditions, such as chronic liver disease or chronic kidney failure. These illnesses are unrelated to fertility but they can affect the whole body, including the reproductive system, upsetting the balance of reproductive hormones and even causing testicular damage and a loss of libido. Although thyroid disease is a rare cause of male infertility, men with an overactive or under-active thyroid are susceptible to fertility problems. The hormonal control of sperm production may be affected by diabetes. There has long been a belief that men with diabetes were less fertile. Research shows that, in fact, their sperm swim in straighter lines than those of non-diabetics, therefore reaching the egg more quickly. Men with diabetes do tend to have other fertility problems, however.

Be sure to ask your doctor or fertility consultant all the questions you have about your condition.

Age also has an impact on hormonal balance in men. This is a major factor affecting fertility and is not just confined to women (see pages 16–17). Men experience what has been termed andropause, which is similar to menopause in women, when hormone levels change and sperm quality may be adversely affected as a result.

Being overweight or taking an excessive amount of physical exercise may also affect hormone levels, as can the amount of stress in your lives and other aspects of your lifestyle (see pages 33–43).

Damage to the testes

If the testes themselves are damaged, the release of the hormones they produce is also affected. As a result, gonadotrophin hormone levels increase to try and compensate. Men with testicular failure either produce no sperm or very few. In some cases, the damage may be so great that there is a complete absence of germ cells from which sperm are derived (Sertoli-cell-only syndrome). Testicular failure may be due to any of a number of reasons.

Genetic defects Klinefelter's syndrome is a genetic condition that results in a man having an extra X-chromosome. This is a leading cause of testicular failure, which can also occur in men who have an extra Y-chromosome. Some genetically normal men (that is, they have XY-chromosomes) produce testosterone, but none of the cells in the body recognize it so the men develop as females. This is known as testicular feminization. In about 6 per cent of men who have permanently low sperm counts (fewer than 5 million per ml), small amounts of the Y-chromosome responsible for the normal functioning of the testes are missing.

Alterations in chromosomes other than the sex chromosomes may also adversely affect male fertility (autosome disorders). These conditions are known as balanced translocations and inversions. In addition, testicular failure may be associated with other problems as a result of a genetic disorder, such as coeliac disease and sickle cell disease.

Birth defects Cryptorchidism, or undescended testes, is a birth defect that frequently leads to testicular failure. Men who have one normal testis are more likely to be fertile.

Inflammation of the testes Known as orchitis, testicular inflammation does not always affect fertility but, at worst, it may lead to a reduction in the release of testosterone and an end to sperm production. Sexually transmitted infections (STIs) such as herpes, syphilis, chlamydia and gonorrhoea are the leading causes of inflammation, as is mumps if it occurs after puberty. Orchitis also occurs with tuberculosis, typhoid and some tropical diseases. In addition, any condition such as influenza, which causes a fever with a temperature of more than 38.5°C (101.3°F), may damage sperm production for up to six months.

Physical traumas Accidents such as a kick in the groin are only likely to damage the testes if the trauma is severe. Twisting of the testis (torsion) can block the blood supply to the testis. If this condition is not treated quickly – within six hours – it can result in permanent damage.

Ejaculation problems

Retrograde ejaculation This occurs when the muscles that pump the semen through the penis do not work properly. Instead, semen is pushed back into the bladder. This condition may be caused by ailments that damage nerves, such as diabetes or paraplegia, and sometimes surgery to remove the prostate. It is possible to recover sperm from your partner's urine, and prepare it for intra-uterine insemination (IUI, see pages 152–53).

Impotence This may be caused by conditions such as diabetes, paraplegia or other diseases of the nervous system, as well as previous surgery that has affected parts of the male reproductive system. In most cases, however, the roots of impotence are of a psychological nature. The problem can usually be treated by means of counselling.

Obstruction Blockages in the male reproductive system may also give rise to infertility, as they do in females. In some cases, surgery such as a hernia repair may result in an obstruction, but by far the most common cause of inflammation and subsequent blockage are sexually transmitted infections (see pages 108–11).

If there are no sperm present in the semen, either your partner is not producing any sperm (non-obstructive azoospermia) or he has a blockage in the reproductive system preventing the sperm from being ejaculated (obstructive azoospermia).

Absence of the vas deferens Some men have no vas deferens, the tubes linking the testes to the penis. This condition is known as congenital bilateral absence of the vas deferens, or CBAVD. It has been associated with cystic fibrosis, so men with CBAVD should be tested for cystic fibrosis to prevent the possibility of them passing it on.

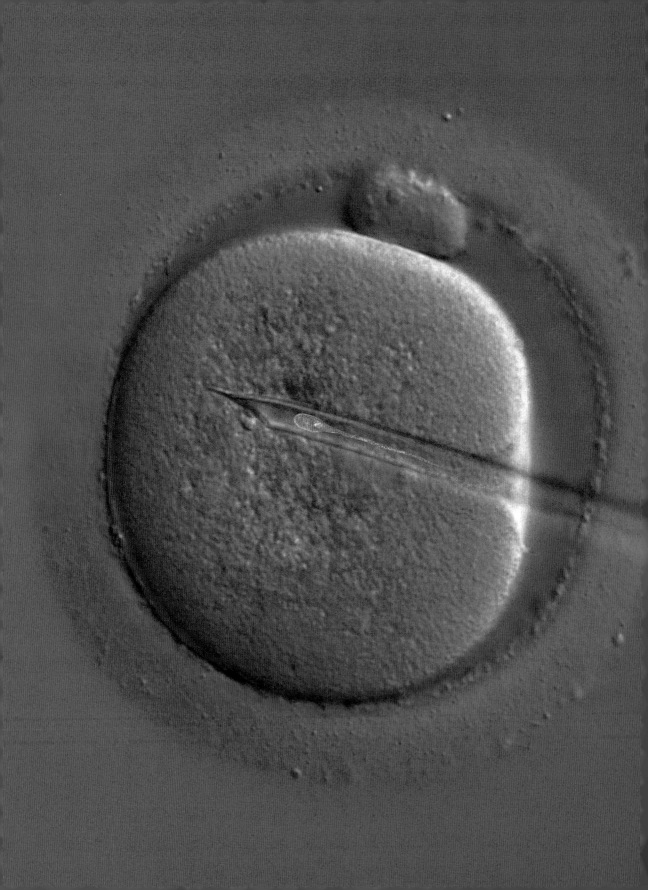

Assisted conception

By now, you will know whether or not you have a fertility problem. You will probably have identified the cause and be considering the use of *assisted reproductive technology* to help you conceive. This chapter describes the *options* that your fertility consultant might offer you; in particular, in vitro fertilization (IVF). Fertility treatment does not have to be a daunting prospect if you prepare yourselves properly, and you can *improve your chances of successful treatment* through an appropriate diet and lifestyle and the use of certain complementary therapies.

Your treatment options

Now that you and your partner have had a variety of fertility tests, you will have a clearer idea of how best to proceed to the treatment stage of Plan B. There is likely to be a range of options for you both to consider in consultation with your clinic.

Weighing everything up

Armed with test results, you will be able to discuss with your doctor or fertility consultant how to adapt the most appropriate treatment for you to suit your particular needs and circumstances, bearing in mind, for example, your age, the specific results of blood tests and your feelings about and reactions to what you have learnt so far about your fertility. Do not agree to proceed with anything that you are not completely happy about and keep doing your own research. The Human Fertilization and Embryology Authority (HFEA) is a good source of information. You might also like to visit websites for information or support (see page 187).

Many couples who discover that they have fertility problems have to consider assisted reproductive techniques (ARTs) – high-technology procedures that bring together sperm and egg. They include in vitro fertilization (IVF), and ICIS and IMSI techniques that use high-powered microscopes to select sperm (see page 174).

Accepting intervention

The thought of intervention in conception may be a daunting prospect. If it is possible, start with less interventionist procedures and build up. No procedure will seem as frightening once you are underway. Where you start, however, will depend upon the results of fertility testing. It might be ovulation induction (OI), intra-uterine insemination (IUI), in vitro fertilization (IVF) or a combination of treatments.

Various treatment protocols are discussed in the pages that follow, in a format that makes it easier for you to understand what will be happening on various days of your cycle, when to take drugs and when you will need an ultrasound scan or a blood test, for example. Procedures may be helped along their way by using complementary remedies and changing aspects of your lifestyle.

Zita's tips

* **Do your research methodically and logically:** after you have received a diagnosis, work out a plan of action, find out exactly what is involved, decide which clinic you would like to attend and calculate how much any treatment is likely to cost.

* **Beware of information overload:** it may seem that everyone is telling you what you should do; which treatment you should have; the best clinic to visit; the latest research you should know about. Others may have sound advice to give you, especially if they have also been through fertility treatment, but remember that your situation is unique, and you and your partner need to take time to find the solutions that are right for you.

* **Stay focused on one thing at a time:** there may be several treatment options to consider. Don't panic and career off in different directions at once.

Complementary therapies

The wealth of complementary therapies available offers varying degrees of help and hope to couples with fertility problems. Although you do need to be realistic about how much these treatments might be able to help, there are many good reasons for giving them a try. Do be wary of some over-enthusiastic therapists, however, making unproven claims and offering false hope.

Setting a time frame

I am a great believer in complementary therapies, but it is important to work within a time frame. Many women choose to go down the route of trying therapy after therapy, and time can pass very quickly. Please do a review of what you are doing every three months.

Choosing a therapy

Choosing to go down the complementary route does not mean forgoing conventional medicine. We are talking "complementary", not "alternative", therapies. Most will help to increase your general state of health by improving the functioning of all your body systems.

There is little hard evidence to support most complementary therapies and few doctors are willing or able to give extensive advice. Unproven doesn't necessarily mean ineffective, however, and there is plenty of anecdotal evidence. Remember that every individual's case is unique and there is no guarantee that what has worked for one person will also have a positive outcome for you.

Find out as much information as you can about all the individual therapies you are considering – from support groups, books, magazines, the library, the internet – before making your choice. Find out how long the treatment has been in use and how widespread it is. Some therapies, such as herbal medicine and acupuncture, have been around for thousands of years. Trust your instincts if you feel particularly drawn to one type of therapy.

Complementary benefits

Most complementary treatments and remedies, while not solving your fertility problems, will contribute to an integrated healthcare plan that will make assisted reproductive techniques more likely to succeed. Complementary therapies provide a range of benefits:

* **a sense of control** and direct involvement in your treatment programme
* **control over who you see** and when you see them
* **sympathetic treatment** that engenders a real sense of being listened to
* **plenty of time to ask questions** and discuss your fertility problems in greater depth
* **holistic treatment** that addresses the mental and emotional as well as the physical aspects of your case
* **a greatly reduced risk of unpleasant** or dangerous side effects
* **physical and emotional support** to help you tolerate the protocols of IVF
* **encouragement to take responsibility** for your own healthcare and treatment programme
* **help with mental and physical relaxation** so that you can cope with stress
* **an opportunity for your partner** to become more involved, depending on the therapy
* **nutritional advice** and recommendations about lifestyle changes to encourage successful treatment
* **improved health generally,** accompanied by an enhanced sense of wellbeing.

There is a great deal of documented research about the benefits of the ancient practice of acupuncture.

feel shy or embarrassed about asking them. Find out how much experience they have in the field of fertility, what training they have had, how long they have been practising, what their fees are and if they are affiliated to the appropriate professional body. Be wary of anyone who makes wild promises or asks for money up front. Trust your instincts. If at any point you feel uneasy or unhappy, say so. If your issues are not addressed satisfactorily, go to another practitioner.

It is important that you do not feel as if you are being controlled by a practitioner and that you like him or her. You must be realistic about your expectations and not develop false hope. This is especially important if your FSH (follicle-stimulating hormone) levels are high or if you are older. You cannot afford to wait very long in hope before going down an interventionist route.

Acupuncture

My own speciality is acupuncture (see pages 72–73) so I'm naturally somewhat biased in its favour. I work closely with doctors and specialists at various clinics and have had a great deal of success in helping women to conceive naturally or supporting them through fertility treatment. There is a great deal of documented evidence on acupuncture and electro-acupuncture. A Swedish study in 1996, for example, established that electro-acupuncture improved uterine blood flow in infertile women. Many studies have shown that it can help to:

* improve male fertility by improving sperm quality – count, concentration and motility
* aid hormonal balance
* relieve symptoms of endometriosis (see page 114)
* induce ovulation in women with polycystic ovary syndrome (PCOS, see page 119)
* regulate the menstrual cycle, especially shortening a long cycle
* improve general health.

Always get a full medical diagnosis first and don't abandon mainstream medicine. Keep your doctor fully informed about which complementary therapies you are having and tell your therapist about any conventional drugs you have been prescribed by your doctor or a fertility consultant. Ideally you should all be able to work together: collaboration is the key.

Choosing a practitioner

As with fertility clinics and specialists, nothing beats the combination of thorough research and personal recommendation. Try to get several word-of-mouth recommendations. Support groups are useful for this, or ask another practitioner whose opinion you value.

Talk to a therapist before committing yourself to a particular course of treatment – it is important to feel confident and comfortable and to establish a good rapport. A good practitioner should be empathetic and receptive to questions, so don't

If you have rejected acupuncture because you are needle phobic, I can tell you that the needles used are very fine – little thicker than a hair – and that the discomfort is minimal.

Chiropractic

Chiropractic has been found to improve fertility, possibly by releasing pressure on the spinal nerves connecting with the uterus. It can also address neck and pelvic problems and hormonal dysfunction caused by a restriction of the sphenoid bone or its membrane attachments, which may affect the functioning of the pituitary gland. The approach is holistic and takes into account posture, lifestyle, diet, work conditions and even the height and hardness of your bed. It is important to find out not only what has gone wrong but why, so that bad habits can be corrected and the problem is less likely to recur. A treatment usually lasts about 45 minutes and is totally safe and non-invasive.

Cranial osteopathy

Cranial treatment may help the pituitary gland to function properly if there is a hormonal imbalance. A treatment usually lasts for about 40 minutes and you may find you feel slightly light-headed for a short while afterwards.

Herbal medicine

Herbs have been used medicinally for thousands of years. The whole of the plant, including the roots, is used, not just the active constituent, so herbs tend to have a much gentler impact on the body than conventional drugs, and they have few unpleasant side effects. Always choose sources of organically grown herbs if you can.

There are a number of herbs that can help with fertility problems, hormone imbalance (see page 131) and specifically female dysfunctions, but I do not recommend that you self-prescribe. Consult a qualified herbalist, preferably with experience in treating women who have fertility problems.

Homeopathy

There are homeopathic remedies to treat both male and female fertility problems. In some cases homeopathic preparations may help to eliminate hormonal imbalance and disorders, correct menstrual irregularities and improve a variety of reproductive functional disorders. Homeopathic remedies are available over the counter at many chemists and health shops, but I would strongly recommend that you have a consultation with a qualified and experienced practitioner to determine the appropriate constitutional remedy for your particular needs. A first appointment can last between one and two hours. Details of your temperament, medical history, habits, likes and dislikes, hopes and fears are noted, allowing the practitioner to build up a complete picture of you and identify the right remedy. Lifestyle changes may be recommended. Symptoms may get slightly worse initially, or old ones briefly resurface, before your condition improves. Once there is a marked improvement

Herbs treat the symptoms but also address the causes of a problem, helping the body back into a state of balance.

you should stop taking the remedy. The number of consultations needed varies from person to person. It is quite safe to take homeopathic remedies whilst being treated with conventional drugs.

Hypnotherapy

Hypnotherapy has gradually gained the respect of the medical establishment. It has had a degree of success in treating some cases of unexplained fertility. It can remove subconscious mental blocks that may be preventing you from conceiving and also help you to relax about the issue of fertility. Stress levels can be reduced by hypnotherapy, and some patients have reported that, as a result, high prolactin levels have also been lowered. Women who have suffered termination, miscarriage, abuse or violence can be helped to let go of the grief and guilt associated with a trauma in their past.

The choice of homeopathic remedy will be based on your constitutional make-up and your specific fertility problem.

Under hypnosis, the conscious part of the brain is temporarily bypassed, allowing the subconscious part, which influences mental and physical functions, to take control. In this state of profound relaxation you are extremely receptive to suggestion, and you can be desensitized as far as phobias and deep-rooted fears are concerned.

Ninety per cent of the population are thought to be capable of entering hypnosis. The state is pleasant and comfortable and, despite myths to the contrary, can only work with your consent, so you always remain in control. If you find it difficult to relax into a meditative state, a hypnotherapist can teach you how to quieten the mind and relax the body for visualization and affirmations, as well as work with you to improve your positive outlook. There are no side effects.

Osteopathy

Osteopathy can help to correct some of the structural problems that lead to infertility by restoring and maintaining balance in the neuro-musculoskeletal systems of the body. There are three main areas of structural and postural strain: the mid-cervical, dorso-lumbar junction and sacroiliac joint. Misuse or trauma can upset the fine balance between muscles, joints, ligaments and nerves, resulting in ovarian and uterine irritation and dysfunction. Osteopathy tries to restore and maintain this balance. There has already been much research in this field, and more investigative projects are underway in the UK using osteopaths within the National Health Service.

Osteopaths assess the whole person and do not just study a condition or its specific symptoms. At your first appointment the practitioner will take a full case history. You'll be asked to undress to your underwear and the osteopath will make detailed observations of your posture, weight distribution, mobility and so on before making a diagnosis and suggesting a treatment plan. Treatment is usually weekly until symptoms improve. There are few side effects, though you may feel tired after a treatment and the symptoms might get worse for 24 hours or so before they get better.

Reflexology

Reflexology is a technique of foot massage. It is used to a lesser extent on the hands. The nerve endings are stimulated by massage to effect changes in other parts of the body; the feet are believed to represent a map of the whole body. Although reflexology is not a diagnostic tool, it may detect signs of disorder or disease. It does not aim to treat illness specifically but to stimulate the body's own ability to rebalance and heal itself. There is little research data on reflexology and fertility but it is a particularly successful treatment for stress relief and relaxation and works well as a "complement" to orthodox treatment.

Treatment can take up to an hour or more and six weekly sessions are usually recommended. The therapist moves his or her thumbs across your feet, covering every minute point, including those corresponding to the ovaries, uterus, hypothalamus and pituitary gland. The aim is to activate the body's self-healing capacity by stimulating the reflex points, or to calm and relax zones where there are indications of acute disturbance.

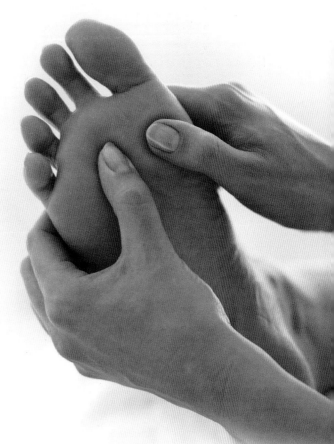

Reflexology is good for stress relief and relaxation.

Lymphatic drainage

This procedure helps to rid the body of toxins by encouraging the action of the lymphatic system. Light pressure is applied to the skin in gentle rhythmic movements that manually assist the flow of lymph. The lymph system is a vitally important part of the immune system – it is, in effect, the body's waste disposal system, clearing away toxins, bacteria and cell debris. If it is not functioning properly, blockages in the waste-disposal system may occur. There are many lymph nodes located in the groin area and clearing these will improve blood supply to the whole pelvic area. A lymphatic drainage session usually lasts for about an hour.

I sometimes suggest lymphatic drainage to some of my clients as part of a fertility treatment programme. It is particularly useful prior to an IVF (in vitro fertilization) cycle or in between other specific courses of fertility treatment.

Any complementary treatment that involves deep breathing techniques or is meditative has a calming effect on the body and helps you to relax and relieve stress. It may also help to build up reserves of energy by focusing your mind and clearing out a lot of the unnecessary "clutter" in your head.

Ovulation induction

Ovulation induction (OI), or ovarian stimulation, is a way of regulating your menstrual cycle by kickstarting ovulation in order to increase your chances of conceiving naturally.

Q&A

* What is the success rate for clomiphene?
Eighty per cent of viable pregnancies that come about following the use of clomiphene occur during the first three months of stimulation. Very few pregnancies occur among women who have taken clomiphene for six months or more without a break.

* How is it taken?
Clomiphine is taken orally (in tablet form), usually for five days each month and starting with a dose of 50mg, on days 2–6 of your cycle. It induces ovulation on day 13 or 14 if you have a regular 28-day cycle. The dosage may be increased to 100mg the following month if you have not ovulated, but doses higher than 150mg are not often recommended. Protocols vary from clinic to clinic.

* Is it an expensive treatment?
Cost varies according to the combinations of drugs used, but is in the hundreds rather than thousands of pounds.

* Are there any side effects?
Some women suffer headaches and nausea, weight gain and bloating. In the event that higher doses than 150mg are necessary, clomiphene may cause hot flushes, breast tenderness or migraines.

* Is there anything I need to do while I am on the treatment?
There is a limited amount of research to suggest that 500mg of vitamin C a day may potentiate the action of clomiphene.

Who is it suitable for?

Ovulation induction is recommended for women whose periods are irregular as a result of an inadequate or unbalanced production of FSH (follicle-stimulating hormone) or LH (luteinizing hormone). These women's ovaries and hormonal systems are functioning, but they need help to ovulate regularly and develop follicles to maturity.

OI is also recommended for women who have polycystic ovary syndrome (PCOS – see pages 119–121) or a luteal phase defect (LPD – see page 128). In the case of the latter, insufficient amounts of progesterone are produced in the luteal phase of the cycle (see pages 10–11). The drug used in OI (see below) enhances progesterone production by making multiple follicles, although there is still some debate about its use for women with an LPD.

How the drugs work

The drug used in OI is clomiphene citrate (brand names Clomid or Serophene). HCG (human chorionic gonadotrophin) injections may also be given (see below). Clomiphene binds to oestrogen receptor sites in the brain, fooling the body into thinking that the amount of oestrogen in the blood is too low. This stimulates the hypothalamus to release more GnRH (gonadotrophin-releasing hormone), prompting the pituitary gland to release more LH and FSH. This causes a follicle to start maturing an egg ready for ovulation.

There is a certain amount of debate about the safety of clomiphene. Apart from the side effects that some women suffer (see box, left), in about

15 per cent of cases too many eggs are produced. This is known as ovarian hyperstimulation. Regular monitoring of women taking this drug is essential. Ultrasound scans check the number and development of follicles in the ovaries. If more than three large follicles are found to have developed, treatment may be suspended because of the increased risk of multiple births.

In addition, clomiphene has a drying effect on cervical secretions and results in a thinning of the endometrium over time, reducing the chances of implantation. The drug should not be given unless tests have shown evidence of an ovulation disorder because of this effect on secretions and it should not be taken for more than six cycles (months). A month's break after three months is advisable – this is important if you are going on to have further treatments. There are links between the prolonged use of clomiphene (a year or more) and ovarian cancer, and the drug is associated with a higher rate of miscarriage. It is important to take the lowest possible dose, but you may be advised that it needs to be increased, of course, depending on your circumstances. Discuss all these potentially worrying issues with your fertility consultant.

Figures show that, after a course of clomiphene, about 80 per cent of women with irregular or no ovulation will ovulate, and about 40 per cent of those who do ovulate will conceive within six months of treatment. Twenty per cent of women have no response to clomiphene; those over the age of 40, in particular, may not respond well to it.

Clomiphene and HCG

If ovulation induction using clomiphene alone has not been successful, the next step may be to have an injection of HCG to encourage the final maturation of the follicle and the release of the egg. This drug is generally administered when one follicle reaches a diameter of at least 18mm (½in). Sexual intercourse or intra-uterine insemination (IUI – see pages 152–53) will be timed for 36–40 hours after the injection has been administered.

Case history

Lee, aged 34, first realized she had a problem at the age of 18, when her periods stopped and then became very erratic. She also found herself losing weight. She married in her early 20s and tried unsuccessfully for a family for 18 months before seeking medical help. **Following a laparoscopy, she was diagnosed with PCOS and was prescribed Clomid.** Treatment was successful and within two months she was pregnant. Lee's periods continued to be erratic following the birth of her son. **When she decided to try for another child 18 months later, she was given Clomid and her second son was born two and a half years after the first.**

A mature ovarian follicle containing a ripe egg.

Intra-uterine insemination

The aim of intra-uterine insemination (IUI), or artificial insemination as the procedure used to be called, is to place active sperm close to an egg to assist fertilization.

Who is it suitable for?

IUI may be the next step for women for whom ovulation induction using clomiphene alone has not been successful. It is a way of assisting natural fertilization when there is a problem with sperm quality, there are reduced numbers of anti-sperm antibodies, FSH (follicle-stimulating hormone) levels are high, or in some cases of unexplained infertility or endometriosis. The procedure is not recommended for women who have blocked Fallopian tubes or whose partners have a very low or non-existent sperm count or poor sperm quality (a minimum of 1 million washed sperm per millilitre is required for this procedure).

How IUI works

After ovulation, a sample of washed sperm is injected directly into the uterus by means of a catheter through the cervix. IUI treatment may involve the use of clomiphene to stimulate the follicles or injections, depending on clinic protocols. Ovulation may be induced by means of an HCG (human chorionic gonadotrophin) injection (see opposite). The procedure is performed as near as possible – ideally within six hours – to ovulation, which is determined by an ultrasound scan or by using an ovulation predictor kit. Two IUIs may be scheduled by some clinics – one just prior to ovulation and the other around ovulation. Protocols will vary from clinic to clinic.

IUI protocol

Days of cycle	1–5 Menstrual period	6–10	11–13
Stage of egg development			
Drugs	* Clomiphene, usually on days 2–6		* HCG injection if needed
Scans, tests and procedures		* Ultrasound scan on day 10 to see if follicles are developing	* Ultrasound scan * Home ovulation kit to detect LH surge to check if ovulating

IUI *with drugs*

With IUI alone, there is a 10 per cent rate of success per cycle. IUI with clomiphene increases this figure to 10–15 per cent. The latter option is usually recommended when the use of clomiphene alone hasn't been successful in a previous attempt. IUI combined with an HCG injection – to encourage follicle maturation and the release of an egg – is another option.

With each stage of IUI treatment, the necessary medications get stronger in order to increase the chances of success. As a consequence of the strength and cost of the drugs involved, however, I do advise choosing the gentlest options first and building up only if you are unsuccessful. Having acupuncture at weekly intervals while you are going through IUI may be of benefit, as may other complementary treatments (see pages 145–49).

I would also recommend that you choose a clinic for IUI treatment that is open at weekends. I have seen many disappointed women who have known they are ovulating during a weekend but have been unable to do anything about it because their clinic has been closed at the time.

Case history

Sandra, aged 35, and her partner tried for a baby for two years before seeking help. Clomid was prescribed, with few side effects, and **Sandra had three IUIs in consecutive months.** The third was successful and Sandra now has a baby boy. *"The procedure was uncomfortable and unpleasant; it was cold and clinical and so far removed from how I imagined my baby would be conceived. Also, the clinic gave me hardly any time to lie down after the procedure, and I've since learned that this is quite important. **So I was amazed and absolutely delighted when it worked – third time lucky!"***

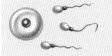
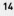

14

* Washed sperm injected into uterus via cervix

Q&A

* **What is the success rate of IUI?**
It's about 10 per cent per cycle but drugs can improve this (see above).

* **How long does it take and is it a painful procedure?**
It takes a few minutes and usually causes little or no discomfort; you may feel wet as a result of the cervix being washed beforehand. Cramping is occasionally felt afterwards.

* **Do I need to rest after having IUI?**
Yes. Clinics generally don't allow you long enough after the procedure. Remain lying down for at least 30 minutes after the procedure and then take it easy for a while.

* **How many IUIs should we try before moving on to IVF?**
In general, three IUIs using clomiphene, followed by three attempts with injections, should bring success. If not, discuss IVF with your clinic. Take your age into account, however. Three cycles of IUI might "delay" you for 4–6 months before moving on to IVF.

In vitro fertilization

Embarking on IVF is a major decision and one that you should not rush into. It requires a great deal of research and thought and then mental and emotional preparation.

Being prepared

You need to be very sure about what you are doing, why you are doing it, the possible effects, the time it will take, the costs involved and the emotional roller coaster you may have to endure. Thinking ahead is very important, and planning your diary is the best preparation you can do.

What is IVF?

IVF stands for in vitro fertilization – in vitro means "in glass". It involves an egg being fertilized in a Petri dish in a laboratory under very carefully controlled conditions.

In a normal, natural cycle, usually only one egg ripens within a growing follicle. The egg is released and, if fertilized (penetrated by a sperm) in one of the Fallopian tubes, it travels to the uterus

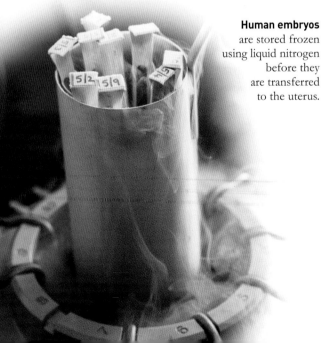

Human embryos are stored frozen using liquid nitrogen before they are transferred to the uterus.

where it implants and grows. With IVF, the aim is to cultivate multiple follicles to harvest many eggs, which are surgically extracted and fertilized outside the body. They are then placed in the uterus, which has been prepared by hormone treatment to be ready to receive an embryo.

Planning your time

There are key stages in the IVF process when you must put aside adequate amounts of time and give priority to the treatment above all your other commitments. In the first week, blood tests and scans may take up time, so plan your diary. Don't be surprised if clinics run late. Bear all this in mind when planning your work schedule for that week. Even when consultations run according to schedule, results may not do so, and you need to be prepared to be called unexpectedly. Discussing the consequences of your results may take time. And do not be surprised if some tests or procedures have to be repeated.

The egg retrieval process doesn't take very long but you may feel some effects afterwards. You may feel groggy, for instance, if you have had an anaesthetic. I always recommend a rest afterwards to allow the body to heal. Following the transfer of embryos rest for at least a day (most women feel this instinctively). Carry out only light duties in order to give implantation the best chance of success.

Deciding who to tell

If you are still working full time, you must face the difficult decision about whether or not to confide in your boss or other colleagues, given that treatment can demand a lot of time out of your working week and you have no guarantees that the treatment will work on the first attempt. My advice would be not to broadcast what you are doing but find a friend in whom you can confide, preferably one who's had a similar experience and who can understand what you are going through.

Thinking it through

The procedures and drugs used in IVF place huge demands on the day-to-day routine for both partners. Some of the risks and side effects, such as irritability, hot flushes and other symptoms, are well documented. The immediate effects of the medication last only as long as you are taking the drugs. It may be some time yet, however, before we become aware of all the long-term health implications of IVF – a possible link has been made, for example, between an increased incidence of certain female cancers and IVF treatment and a new register has been set up to gather data.

Doing research

Discuss the IVF route thoroughly with your partner and medical advisers, and be sure to take into account your medical history and that of your family – particularly close female relatives. Use every means at your disposal to find out what the latest research and contra-indications may be, since new information is emerging all the time. There are plenty of websites and support groups out there (see page 187) that can provide you with invaluable information.

You may, of course, come across alarming reports during your research, such as the claims about IVF babies having a higher incidence of genetic conditions or abnormalities and being at a greater risk of cancer than naturally conceived children. Discuss any worries that you have with your fertility specialist.

Key considerations

Think long and hard before answering these important questions and make sure you do so with total honesty.

✳ **Can I change my day-to-day routine to make enough time in my life to meet the demands of this treatment?**
Do not underestimate the impact that treatment will have on your, and your partner's, normal routines.

✳ **Will I get the support I need physically, emotionally and mentally from my partner?**
You both need to understand the commitment involved, not just procedurally while you are undergoing tests and treatments, but also when you have to take essential rest at certain key points in the cycle. When I point this out to my female clients, they often say to me, "I wish you would tell my partner that".

✳ **Can I make time not just for the treatment but for other important aspects of life?**
Remember that you have to have a relationship at the end of all of this, whether or not you have a baby.

✳ **How will we get through if I am very stressed?**
Each of you will react in your own way to the problems that IVF treatment throws up along the way. The direct experience that each of you has will be different, and the way in which each of you reacts to your experience may well be different, too. Accept this and get used to the idea now in order to avoid conflict later.

✳ **Do I need another family member or friend in whom I can confide – particularly someone who has gone through the process herself?**
You will need a lot of support while you are undergoing IVF, particularly if your partner finds it hard to cope with all the ups and downs, or he is unable to be there at important moments. It may be useful at times to have the perspective of someone who isn't directly involved.

Getting ready to go

If you have weighed up all the pros and cons and are ready to go ahead with IVF, you must begin to prepare yourself physically and mentally well in advance. This will increase your chance of success so that the number of cycles you may need can be kept to a minimum.

Deciding when to start

Age is one of the key factors in the success of IVF, and you should bear this in mind as you decide when to start the treatment. Unless you have already had preliminary fertility tests carried out, your chosen clinic will need to investigate the reason why you have not conceived in order to plan the right course of treatment for you. Consider having the necessary investigations done in consultation with your clinic or doctor while you are waiting for an appointment to start IVF.

Whatever decisions you make and whatever the eventual outcome of those decisions, you need to be able to look back without regret. Once IVF has begun, you will probably find that the treatment is not as bad as you had anticipated. You will quickly become familiar with the regime of blood tests, scans, nasal sprays and self-injection that treatment involves. I never cease to be amazed at how quickly women acquire detailed knowledge about every aspect of the process. You may know nothing when you first start out, but I promise you that you'll soon be an expert. This knowledge is important because it increases how much control you feel you have over what is happening to you. Men on the whole do not tend to gather as much information as their partners.

Choosing the right clinic

Research, research, research! I cannot overstress the importance of doing your homework before you select a clinic if you choose to go privately. Some people put more effort into choosing a holiday than their IVF clinic. Research will save you time, money and heartache. Word-of-mouth is important but do not rely solely on this – what is right for one couple may not be right for you. Also, IVF techniques are constantly changing, so their experience may be out of date.

Neither should you depend exclusively on your doctor's recommendations. Treatments can vary enormously from clinic to clinic, and where you go may make all the difference to your success. Many clinics have open days and evenings. Canvas the views of other fertility professionals.

Only if your local health authority is funding your

Your chances of success

The pregnancy rate per treatment cycle is about 30 per cent. The clinic you choose can affect the outcome of treatment, and you are likely to respond better at your first attempt. **In addition, your chances will be greater if:**

* you, the female partner, are under the age of 40
* at least one ovary is responding to the stimulation drugs
* your FSH (follicle-stimulating hormone) level is 10 or less (see page 164) on days 2–3 of your cycle and oestradiol, prolactin and LH (luteinizing hormone) levels are at their optimum (see pages 99–100)
* you have had a pregnancy in the past
* your partner has healthy sperm.

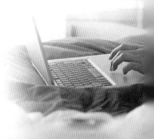

Knowledge is key – it increases your participation in the process and makes you feel more in control.

treatment (that is, NHS treatment) will your choice be limited. They may well be contracted to a particular clinic. If you are paying for your treatment, the choice is all yours. Making the right choice is more important than worrying about offending people. So, if you feel you're at the wrong clinic or that another clinic can offer you something better, don't hesitate to move.

Asking questions

Contact at least two clinics and compare what they have to offer. Read their information packs, decide what your priorities are and draw up a list of questions. Look carefully at costs, which vary enormously. Price should not be the over-riding factor but multiple IVF cycles can be very expensive. Talk to the staff. Feel free to ask anything you think is important. Never feel that a question is trivial or inappropriate. You'll be in contact with your clinic several times a week so find out the name of the person you'll be talking to and how available nurses and doctors are to take calls and answer questions.

I strongly recommend you look at the Human Fertilization and Embryology Authority website – www.hfea.gov.uk – for their guidelines on clinics, and www.fertilityfriends.co.uk for first-hand support or feedback, such as their success rates, from other couples undergoing IVF. The internet is also a valuable source of information about assisted reproductive techniques used abroad that may be relevant to your treatment but not available in this country. Getting treatment abroad can be very expensive but your specialist may be able to incorporate certain aspects into your own protocol.

Assessing a clinic

* **Location** – be prepared to put yourself out to get to a clinic that has a particularly good reputation.

* **Opening hours** – choose a clinic that is available seven days a week if necessary.

* **Reputation and success rates** – what are the statistics for your age, particular fertility problem, etc.?

* **Specialist expertise** – do they treat older women, those who have high FSH levels or those who have had multiple IVF failures or recurrent pregnancy loss?

* **Reviews after failed cycles** – check if these are included in the basic price for the IVF cycle.

* **Are the appropriate treatments** to suit your particular requirements available?

* **What is the level of general care:** do the staff put you at ease? Will they be accessible if you have questions or concerns?

* **Availability of counselling** – some clinics have a better reputation for providing counselling than others (see box, page 158).

* **Waiting times** – bear in mind that it may be worth going on the waiting list of your chosen clinic in advance of when you want to start treatment.

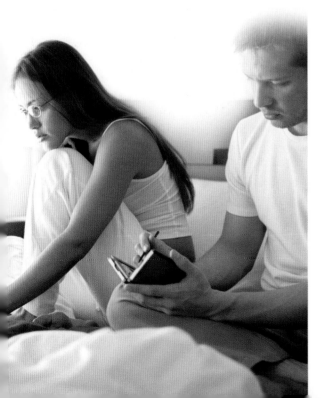

Meeting your consultant

Having researched and chosen your clinic, you will meet your consultant to discuss in detail your medical and surgical history and any previous fertility treatments, and to talk about and decide upon the appropriate course of action for you.

Clinics are legally obliged to collect certain information (names, dates of birth, medical details), which is passed on to the Human Fertilization and Embryology Authority (HFEA) and held on its computer register. The information is confidential.

Before treatment begins, you and your partner have to, by law, give your written consent. Do this only when you are satisfied that you understand completely the details and implications of what you are agreeing to. The special HFEA consent forms include your agreement to:

* The storage of any gametes or embryos created for your future use. Also, you may choose to allow them to be used in research or to donate them.

Counselling

All licensed UK clinics must offer you counselling before treatment starts. You don't have to accept but it can provide a useful opportunity to discuss any concerns you have. The quality of counselling varies enormously. The HFEA code of practice sets out the various types, which include:

IMPLICATIONS COUNSELLING
To consider ethical issues. This is especially helpful for those considering the use of donated sperm, eggs or embryos or surrogacy. It may also include genetic counselling.

SUPPORT COUNSELLING
To give emotional support, especially if treatment fails.

THERAPEUTIC COUNSELLING
To help couples to cope with their fertility problems and the consequences of tests and treatment, to adjust their expectations and accept their situation.

* The procedures of treatment, such as egg collection and embryo transfer, and the disclosure of identifying information to your doctor or, for example, the HFEA, who may need to know details for their records or research.

Screening for infections

There are a number of routine tests (blood tests and swabs) to check for infections before any IVF cycle can begin. Following positive tests, antibiotics will be prescribed. You will be re-tested two weeks later to see if you are free of infection.

Chlamydia (see page 110) This causes inflammation, and perhaps even permanent damage, to the Fallopian tubes.

Ureaplasma (see Bacterial vaginosis, page 112) This is a micro-organism that does not normally cause symptoms, which can be present in either partner and may interfere with implantation.

HIV In the UK, only a few hospitals are currently prepared to accept people for IVF treatment if they test positive for the HIV virus.

Heptatitis B and C Many clinics will not allow you to proceed with IVF treatment if you test positive for hepatitis.

Rubella Exposure to rubella during pregnancy may cause birth defects in the baby. If you do not have rubella antibodies, you need to be immunized before embarking on IVF. You will be rechecked for immunity a few months later.

Thinking positively

Try to enter every treatment cycle with a positive attitude. Think of IVF, as with all assisted reproductive techniques, as a course of treatment. Be realistic about your chances and keep your feet firmly on the ground, but don't give up if you don't meet with success straight away. IVF doesn't work for everyone but there is a great deal you can do yourself to improve your chances of success.

Write a list of positive affirmations and repeat them to yourself every day:
* My body is healthy and able to grow and sustain a pregnancy.
* I accept each stage of this process and believe that it will have the best possible outcome.
* Everything is working as it should be and going according to plan.

Always bear in mind that the IVF process is taking you closer to your goal of having a baby. Don't be overwhelmed by any one stage, test result or consultation, and constantly keep an eye on what will hopefully be the end result.

It is important to keep communicating with your partner and offering each other mutual support. It is all too easy to allow the stresses of treatment to come between you, particularly if you have different ways of dealing with things. Not all men will share their partner's obsession with researching the finer points of treatment, while others will read the technical manuals in order to avoid dealing with the emotional implications.

I have seen some women grow increasingly frustrated with what they perceive to be their partner's lack of understanding of and commitment to the IVF treatment programme, while others go overboard trying not to overburden their partner with their concerns. It is important to recognize that IVF may be tough for you but it can also be a really difficult time for your partner as well. He may feel frustrated, powerless, even guilty, as he watches you taking medication and undergoing the various procedures. Find out if he wants to become more involved in the process, perhaps by helping you with the injections or accompanying you to scans. If he doesn't want to, try not to take it personally and, whatever you do, don't put him under pressure to do what doesn't come naturally.

Considering costs

* **My husband and I are wondering how we'll pay for IVF. What costs should we budget for?**
Most fertility clinics, including centres in university and NHS hospitals, are wholly fee-paying, but the costs may vary hugely from clinic to clinic. You need to find out exactly what the charges are, what they include and whether the cost of a treatment cycle (each attempt at achieving a pregnancy) includes items such as drugs, blood tests, scans or sperm, egg and embryo storage.

If you have private medical insurance, find out if it will fund any part of the investigations or treatment. Also, check if any of the fee is refundable by the clinic if a treatment cycle has to be abandoned for any reason.

* **What if we can't afford IVF? Are there any ways of making savings?**
There are no bargains to be had. Some clinics operate within the National Health Service, offering free treatment to patients sponsored by their local health authority. Each LHA decides what funding to allocate to infertility treatment, the types of treatment on offer and eligibility criteria for funding. Some fund drugs for a limited number of cycles. Infertility Network UK may also be able to help (see page 187). Clinical trials, egg-sharing schemes and bursaries are worth investigating. Find out about them on the internet or through the HFEA.

Avoiding time limits

Don't set yourself time limits at the outset – this will make you feel under even more pressure. Take the treatment programme one step at a time and keep reviewing the situation, being prepared to change course (even clinic) as circumstances change. Keep focusing on the positive; if at first you don't succeed, your fertility specialist will have gained a great deal of information that will help fine-tune your treatment in any subsequent cycles. Always ensure that you review each failed cycle to see what can be learned and reworked next time.

Your body and IVF

IVF is a highly technical procedure, so it is easy to feel that you are merely the object of a scientific process and have little influence on that process or the outcome. There is, however, a great deal you can do physically and mentally to minimize side effects and enhance treatment, and to help your body to recover afterwards.

Taking control

The art and science of IVF have been really perfected over the last five years, with often great results. Age, however, will ultimately have the biggest impact on whether it is successful or not.

The procedures and drugs of IVF will place huge demands on your body. To give yourself the best chance of success, start to prepare physically at least 4–6 weeks before treatment begins.

There is a great deal that you can do to help the process along and to give yourself a greater sense of control over the course of events. When I assist women about to undergo IVF, I prepare them mentally, physically and emotionally, offering appropriate help and advice at each stage of the treatment. Some of them have had bad experiences previously, but if you are prepared and focused you can cope with anything and make the most of every experience. Much of the fear and anxiety you might have can be alleviated by understanding how IVF makes use of the body's natural processes, the particular objectives of each stage

of the treatment and the possible results. Use this knowledge to strengthen your natural resources and to help visualize a successful programme.

Preparing the body

Prepare yourself physically for the months of treatment ahead by doing the following:

* If you have already been through one cycle of IVF, you should ideally allow your ovaries to recover for a month or two before embarking on another treatment programme.

* Keep a check on your weight – IVF will have a better chance of success if you are not overweight (see page 29). Most clinics will not accept you if your BMI is over 30 (see page 29). If you are overweight, improve your eating habits so that you lose weight gradually, without depriving yourself of vital nutrients.

* Similarly, if you are significantly underweight, reassess your diet so you can gain the weight you need steadily and healthily.

* Do not smoke and avoid smoky atmospheres – smoking damages the lining of the uterus.

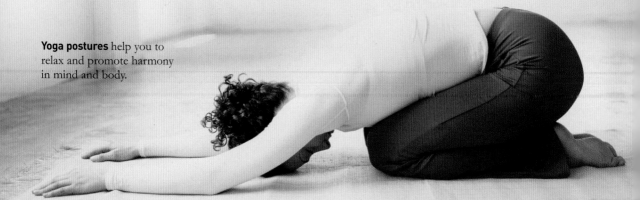

Yoga postures help you to relax and promote harmony in mind and body.

* Try to avoid strenuous exercise, such as aerobics. Your body needs rest as your hormonal system shuts down to prepare for IVF. Take gentle forms of exercise instead, such as walking or yoga.

The importance of good nutrition

Maintaining a healthy diet and following a detox programme can help to fortify body systems that will come under the most stress during IVF. A good dietary practice to start with is to avoid chocolate, sugary and processed foods, salty snacks, coffee, tea, cola drinks and other fizzy drinks and alcohol. These all counteract the beneficial effects of vital nutrients and some have a diuretic effect.

Taking supplements

If you have already been trying to conceive for a while, you and your partner may already be taking nutritional supplements. If not, invest in the best-quality preconception multivitamins and minerals that you can afford (see pages 59–64). Start taking them at least three or four months before your IVF treatment commences. Be wary of some of the anecdotal advice found on internet bulletin boards. This has led some women to take excessive amounts of certain vitamins and minerals. It is worth seeking the advice of nutritional experts.

* Vitamin B-complex: will help your body cope with the stress of invasive procedures.
* Vitamin C: 500mg a day will help collagen production and is vital for wound healing following egg retrieval. There is some evidence to suggest that it may help to prevent miscarriage.
* Vitamin E: enhances healing.
* Zinc: promotes cell formation and wound healing after any surgery and is also vital for hormone production and implantation. Many of the women who come to see me because they have fertility problems are deficient in zinc. This is especially likely if they have been taking the contraceptive pill over a long period of time.
* Inositol: may help to balance blood sugar chemicals in the body.

Zita's tips

I believe it is as important to prepare your body in the run-up to a cycle of IVF treatment as it is to prepare it in anticipation of natural conception. There are a number of measures you might like to consider.

* **A 7- or 10-day detox programme** (see pages 50–53) will help to clear out your system and boost the liver's detoxifying capacity. So, if you have a few weeks before beginning an IVF cycle, spend one of them doing a detox programme.

* **Certain vitamins and other nutrients,** such as vitamin C, vitamin E, selenium, bioflavonoids and glutathione (an amino acid), also help to optimize liver function and protect it from the effects of toxins by increasing the rate at which it processes them. (See pages 59–63 for good food sources of these key nutrients.)

* **Make sure that you take a good multivitamin and mineral** supplement. It should contain magnesium, selenium and zinc. Also consider taking a vitamin C supplement (500mg a day), which will help to replenish the ovaries.

* **Drink** lots of water (see page 58).

* **Consider having a course** of lymphatic drainage (see page 149).

* **Sleep or rest** as much as you can in the weeks leading up to the start of your IVF programme, in order to build up your reserves of energy. You are certainly going to need lots of physical and mental energy to keep you going during the months to come.

* **Spend 20 minutes a day** practising deep breathing techniques (see pages 42–43) and visualization (see pages 43 and 163).

Zita's tips

* **Drink a minimum of 2 litres (3.5 pints) of water** (filtered or still glass-bottled) a day. This should be in addition to other fluids you drink, including herbal teas. Water is vitally important for every cell in the body and to ensure the drugs you take during IVF go where they need to in the body.

* **One of the effects of dehydration** is to switch off the thirst signal in the brain. It is no good starting to drink just before you begin IVF procedures. It's a bit like pouring water on to a parched plant – the water will run straight out of the bottom of the pot without being absorbed. Your body needs time to become properly hydrated.

A good supply of essential nutrients is vitally important in preparation for IVF to support your body's ability to:
* develop mature follicles and eggs
* establish the lining of the uterus
* heal after the retrieval of eggs
* implant an embryo following transfer.

Egg quality will become one of your overriding concerns during the course of your treatment. Make sure you eat plenty of:
* Protein: studies have shown that insufficient amounts of protein in the diet can result in a reduced number of eggs. So you should make sure you eat about 70g (2.5oz) of protein a day (see also pages 55–56). The best-quality protein foods, in terms of amino-acid balance, include eggs, meat, fish, beans, lentils and quinoa. Avoid eating too many dairy products (since milk contains artificial hormones) and eat only organic meat.
* Vitamins and minerals: take a good-quality multivitamin and mineral supplement daily. Studies have also shown that in women on supplementation, the fluid surrounding and nourishing the eggs is rich in vitamins C and E. Zinc, magnesium, selenium and vitamin A are all vital nutrients for egg production, selenium and magnesium have been shown to improve fertilization rates, and folic acid is also important.
* Essential fatty acids: these are vitally important (see pages 63–64). I put all my clients on a DHA supplement in the period leading up to the start of their IVF programme and increase the dosage once stimulation treatment has begun.

Egg retrieval and other invasive techniques used in the IVF programme are regarded as minor surgical procedures, but you need to recover and heal quickly so that you will be ready to receive the embryos shortly afterwards.
* Vitamin C and zinc: take vitamin C (500mg) and zinc (20mg) daily for at least two weeks before the procedure.
* Arnica: this homeopathic remedy may help prevent damage to internal tissues. Consult a practitioner or take the remedy four times daily (6c potency) from the day before retrieval until after the transfer of embryos into the uterus.

The endometrium needs to be about 10mm (½in) thick to receive the embryo and facilitate implantation. The following measures may help to build it up:
* Eat foods that are rich in vitamins B1 and B6. The latter is needed for the production of progesterone and hence the development of the uterine lining. You should also have good intakes of iron and co-enzyme Q10, which is excellent for improving blood flow generally. These vitamins and minerals will help to support and enrich the endometrium. (For good food sources of these nutrients, see pages 60–63).
* The use of acupuncture on certain points on the back has been shown to be of benefit to the uterine lining and to improve pelvic blood flow.

* Drink plenty of water every day.
* Avoid vigorous exercise.
* Use a hot-water bottle to keep the abdomen warm and assist healing.

Acupuncture and IVF

You may find acupuncture treatments beneficial as you prepare for IVF and during the procedures themselves. There are research findings to suggest that acupuncture on a weekly basis may help to build up the lining of the uterus, develop follicles and, after the transfer of embryos, encourage implantation and the maintenance of a pregnancy.

I really believe that, in accordance with traditional Chinese beliefs (see pages 72–73), if your lower abdomen is cold to the touch you should apply warmth to improve your chances of conception. In addition, the kidneys and the liver are considered to be very important for reproduction. The liver is associated with anger, frustration and irritability. Women often complain of experiencing these emotions when they are taking IVF drugs, so encouraging a healthy liver may help to improve the way you feel during your treatment cycle. Acupuncture at certain key points on the liver meridian will help to improve the flow of blood and life energy (*qi*) to a woman's reproductive organs. Treatment of acupoints along the kidney meridian may also help to restore energy depleted during IVF treatment.

Positive visualization

At each stage of your IVF treatment, I want you to visualize what you want to be happening in your body – the eggs maturing, the lining of the uterus thickening, the embryos implanting.

The Chinese believe that if you focus your mind on a particular area in the body, life energy will flow to that spot. Write descriptions of these positive visualizations on cards and place them at points around the house so that you are reminded to repeat them out loud regularly throughout the day. Add other positive affirmations (see page 159)

as well as some statements about how well your body is responding to the drugs and processing them. You may feel a little eccentric doing this, but remember that the mind is an incredibly powerful tool. What you believe shapes what you become. You need to really believe that you are going to have a baby and that in the course of doing so you will remain healthy and not compromise your immune system.

Deep breathing techniques

Breathing slowly, deeply and smoothly (see pages 42–43) can be of great benefit if your stress levels are high and you are emotionally tightly wound. Relaxing your body, encouraging life energy to flow freely and calming your mind will equip you well for the ups and downs of IVF treatments.

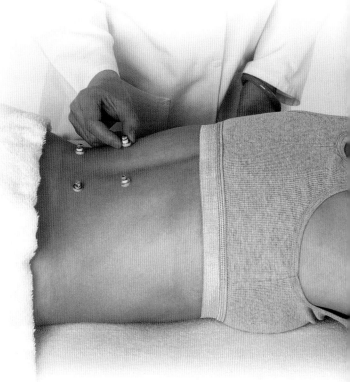

Moxa cones may be placed on kidney and spleen acupoints to encourage the flow of energy and thus improve the chances of conception and reduce the risk of miscarriage.

FSH and IVF

Many women are unable to start IVF treatment because their levels of follicle-stimulating hormone (FSH) are too high. They feel as if they have fallen at the first hurdle and are disappointed, faced with the prospect of putting life on hold as they wait for levels to fall.

The importance of FSH
FSH is the hormone released by the pituitary gland that causes eggs to ripen and mature. If your FSH levels are beyond the expected range, your eggs are likely to be of poor quality. They are much less likely to result in a healthy embryo and consequently a pregnancy.

There are several reasons why you might have raised levels of follicle-stimulating hormone (see pages 128–29). In some cases levels may be low enough to embark on an IVF cycle. Some clinics will begin even if your FSH is relatively high, but the success rate for women who have raised levels is not as good as for those whose levels are normal.

In recent years, AMH (anti-mullerian hormone) blood tests have been used as a good indicator of ovarian reserve (see page 16) and how you are likely to respond to IVF. This test is done in conjunction with an antral follicle count (AFC) scan to check the number of antral follicles on both ovaries.

If your FSH levels are raised, it is important not to put yourself under pressure and increase your stress levels. I often suggest to my clients that they take a break from testing in order to relax. Finding out that your levels are high can be devastating. Explore all the options open to you as a result before deciding whether or not to move on to the next step.

Lowering levels
There is currently no conventional treatment for raised FSH levels. There is some research to suggest that acupuncture may be of benefit, especially using acupoints to help balance the pituitary gland. I treat a number of important points for reproduction and hormone regulation, usually

Interpreting FSH *levels*

DAY-3 FSH (PG/ML)	INTERPRETATION
Less than 6	Excellent result. Very reassuring level.
6–8	Normal. Expect a good response to stimulation.
8–10	Fair. Response is likely to be between normal and slightly reduced (though it will vary widely).
10–12	Lower than normal ovarian reserve. Likely to be a reduced response to stimulation and a reduction in egg and embryo quality with IVF. There are also reduced live birth rates.
12–17	Generally indicates a more marked reduction in response to stimulation and further reduction in egg and embryo quality with IVF. Low live birth rates.
More than 17	Very poor or no response to stimulation. No live births. "No go" levels will be determined by the particular laboratory analysis and IVF centre.

during the last two weeks of a woman's cycle.

Other measures that may help bring levels down:

* Put yourself on a detox programme (see pages 50–53), by drinking plenty of still bottled or filtered water a day, reducing salt intake and avoiding coffee, tea and sugary, carbonated drinks. Try drinking hot water with lemon juice instead.
* Take gentle exercise and, if you are overweight, try to lose weight.
* Spend time relaxing, practising deep breathing or meditating on the colour blue.
* Take B-complex and zinc supplements (see pages 59–63).
* Keep the lower abdomen warm.
* Take an essential fatty acid supplement (see pages 63–64).
* Include beans, pulses, onions and garlic in your diet to help the liver break down oestrogen, and cabbage to increase the rate at which the liver converts oestrogen into its water-soluble form so that it can be excreted. In addition, eating foods that are good sources of phyto-oestrogens (see page 31), such as alfalfa sprouts and linseeds, pulses, oats, parsley, broccoli and Brussels sprouts may also help to correct hormonal imbalance.

Age and egg quality

While an abnormal result (which means high-baseline FSH) tends to be indicative of poor egg quality, a measurement within the expected range does not necessarily mean that the quality of your eggs is good. There are significant numbers of women with normal-baseline FSH values who have poor egg quality that is not being reflected in their FSH reading. This is particularly true of women in their 40s.

An infertile 44-year-old woman with normal FSH (for example, 6) still has a very low probability of conceiving as a result of using IVF, or any other assisted reproductive technique for that matter. It is the fact that she is 44 that diminishes her chances. This is, of course, why IVF programmes have age limits. These restrictions vary from clinic to clinic, but most of them have an age cut-off of between 42 and 45. Older women who have fertility problems will rarely be successful using their own eggs. However, women in their 40s with raised FSH levels may have IVF treatment and consider using donor eggs.

Spend time relaxing, using deep breathing techniques and perhaps meditation or visualization.

IVF protocols

There are two main procedures, or protocols, but the details differ from one clinic to another. Your circumstances will determine which is for you; your response may deviate from the generalized descriptions below.

Who follows which protocol?

The long protocol is for women whose hormones are functioning normally and who have regular cycles. The short protocol is for those who have high FSH (follicle-stimulating hormone) levels or who have responded poorly to ovarian stimulation before.

The long protocol

In this protocol, the body's natural production of FSH and luteinizing hormone (LH) is suppressed or "down-regulated". The cycle is then carefully controlled with drugs to stimulate the ovaries so that many eggs can be produced and harvested.

Long and short IVF protocols

Different clinics have their own protocols and use different drug regimes. This is a basic and generalized illustration.

	LONG PROTOCOL (LP)		LONG PROTOCOL (LP) AND SHORT PROTOCOL (SP)	
Stage	Menstruation	Down-regulation	Menstruation/stimulation	Stimulation continues
Day of cycle	2/3	21–31/33	2–5	6–10
Stage of follicle development				
Treatment and procedures		✳ Suppression drug.	✳ LP: (days 3, 4 or 5) FSH + suppression drug. ✳ SP: (day 2) suppression drug; (day 3) FSH.	✳ Possible FSH adjustments + suppression drug.
Tests and scans	✳ Blood test to check levels of FSH, LH and oestradiol.		✳ LP: suppression check on day 3. Scan to check for cysts and/or blood test to check oestradiol and possibly other hormone levels.	✳ Scans to check progress of follicle development and check thickening of the endometrium. ✳ Blood tests to check oestradiol levels.

You may be given a blood test on day two or three of your menstrual cycle to check levels of FSH, LH and oestradiol (see pages 99–100). If these hormones are at their optimum levels (see box on page 101), you will be able to start the long protocol on day 21 of your cycle.

Down-regulation

At the beginning of a natural ovarian cycle, gonadotrophin-releasing hormone (GnRH) is released into the blood from the hypothalamus in the brain. It is only active for a few seconds but this is sufficient to stimulate the pituitary gland to release FSH, which in turn stimulates several follicles that have begun to develop to continue their growth (see page 10). Under the long protocol, you will be given drugs that have a similar effect to GnRH but remain active in your system for longer than would occur naturally, over-stimulating the pituitary gland so that, in effect, it releases all of its FSH and LH. As levels of these hormones fall, the follicles "recruited" for this cycle do not receive enough hormones to enable them to continue their development. This suppression of the reproductive system wipes the slate clean, so to speak, so that it can begin to be manipulated. The suppression drugs are administered either by injection or nasal spray.

Follicles ripe	Eggs mature	Egg retrieval	Fertilization	Transfer of embryos
11	12	13	14	15–18
* Possible HCG, depending on scan + blood test results.		* Vaginal ultrasound probe or laparoscopy to collect eggs.	* IVF or ICSI method of fertilization. * Grading of embryos .	* Embryos loaded into catheter and inserted into uterus through cervix. * Progesterone or HCG.
* Final scan.				

Checking suppression

Suppression takes 10–12 days; your period should arrive 7–9 days later. Your clinic will schedule a suppression check (ultrasound scan to see if there are any follicular cysts and/or blood test to measure oestradiol levels) on day three of your period. What is considered a "normal" oestradiol level varies from one clinic to another. If the scan detects no cysts and oestradiol levels are down, you are ready to move on to the next stage of the procedure.

Ovarian stimulation

In the next stage of the long protocol treatment, the recruited follicles (see page 10) are stimulated to grow by means of injections of FSH (follicle-stimulating hormone) or FSH and LH (luteinizing hormone) combined. In a natural cycle, the release of FSH is controlled by the pituitary gland so that there is only sufficient to stimulate the largest follicle to ripen fully. In a stimulated cycle, almost all the recruited follicles get that chance.

Q&A

* **How do I know if the drugs are working?**
  You only find out when you have a blood test to check your hormone levels after suppression.

* **How do I know if I am using a nasal spray properly?**
  You will receive instructions from the clinic on the use of a spray. Most women don't have any problems, although it may feel different each time you inhale. Check with your clinic if you are in doubt.

* **What side effects can I expect from the suppression drugs?**
  Different women respond in different ways: some are very sensitive to the medication, while others hardly feel any effects at all. If you are concerned, contact your doctor. Common side effects include:
  * mood swings/emotional fragility
  * irritability and bad temper
  * tiredness
  * hot flushes and sweats
  * breast tenderness
  * vaginal dryness

  * flu-like aches or headaches
  * changes in sex drive
  * irregular bleeding.

* **Should I get my period while on the suppression drugs?**
  Yes, your period will usually arrive 7–9 days after you start taking the drugs. Most clinics will wait until your period starts before commencing stimulation drugs.

* **What if a period doesn't come?**
  Either your system has not shut down yet or you were pregnant before treatment began. Some women do become pregnant by chance while taking the down-regulation drugs and your clinic will test to rule out this possibility.

* **What if my system has not shut down?**
  Usually when this happens a follicle is left over from a previous cycle, or hormone levels are not what your doctor wants them to be. You will have to re-bleed and a drug will be given to start this process. Such a delay will be

discouraging. I have found acupuncture may help to start the bleed.

* **What can go wrong at this stage?**
  Not everybody responds to the suppression drugs. Sometimes, oestradiol levels remain high. The most common problem is an ovarian cyst revealed on an ultrasound scan.

* **What if I have a cyst?**
  Some women are prone to cysts or they may be exacerbated by the drugs. Instead of bursting, as they do in normal ovulation, follicles fill with fluid and oestrogen is produced, interfering with FSH and oestradiol levels. Cysts are not dangerous, although they may be painful.

* **How will the cysts be treated?**
  Some clinics allow you to stay on the suppression medication for a while to see if the cyst disappears on its own. Some clinics will want to remove or drain the cyst before continuing, while others will keep you on the cycle to see if oestradiol levels fall.

You will have injections, at timed intervals during the day, starting on days 3–5 of your period. The drugs used will depend on your particular body chemistry. Some are pure FSH, while others are a combination of FSH and LH. Your doctor will decide which is the most suitable for you. Every woman responds differently to the drugs, some only needing a low dosage while others need more to achieve the same effect.

You will also continue to take suppression drugs in order to maintain a delicate hormonal balance that will allow eggs to ripen but prevent ovulation from occurring before the clinic has a chance to retrieve your eggs. You will continue to take both stimulation and suppression drugs, with possible dosage adjustments, until the eggs are ready to be retrieved (see page 173).

Monitoring your progress

Your progress should be closely monitored. Ultrasound scans of the ovaries and blood tests to measure hormone levels will determine how the follicles are developing. Your doctor will also measure the thickness of the endometrium (by means of ultrasound scanning): 8–10mm (⅓–⅜in) is the optimum. Depending on how your body is responding, drug dosage will be adjusted (within a range of 150–450mg, although sometimes it will be higher than this). Some clinics recommend higher dosages for older women.

If possible, take your partner along with you when you go for a scan, or at least make sure you talk to him on the phone. You may feel the need to discuss the results and their implications with him there and then. Alternatively, you might like to take a friend with you for support in case you hear slightly less-than-positive results from your doctor.

Egg maturation

Around day nine of your cycle, a final scan will check the number and size of follicles and a blood test will check hormone levels, determining when you should have an injection of human chorionic

Zita tips

* **Most women cannot** realistically take the whole time off work during suppression, but be aware of what is happening to your hormonal system and take things as easy as you possibly can. Go with the flow of your body and relax as much as possible.

* **Avoid all aerobic exercise.** I advise all my clients to avoid strenuous exercise. While the reproductive system is shutting down during suppression, they should follow suit. During stimulation while the body is growing eggs, aerobic exercise will take away from this by redirecting blood flow away from the follicles.

* **Sleep is very important:** get plenty of early nights.

* **Keep the lower abdomen warm** to improve the flow of blood in the pelvis.

* **Drink plenty of water** – filtered or still bottled.

* **Spend time alone** if you feel like it; being a bit self-indulgent can do no harm.

* **Acupuncture may help** during the stimulation process.

* **Make sure your diet** includes lots of protein and oily fish such as salmon. I recommend a supplement of evening primrose oil plus DHA. Amino acids are also important. Vitamin C will help to replenish the ovaries. Vitamin E is necessary for the maintenance of cell membranes. (For good food sources of these essential nutrients, see pages 59–64.)

* **If you suffer from headaches,** gently rub lavender oil into your temples.

* **Meditation and visualization** will help you to relax (see page 43). Surround yourself with the colours indigo and blue. Burn lavender oil and focus on the middle of your forehead (the site of the pituitary gland). Visualize your ovaries shutting down.

gonadotrophin (HCG). The injection will be timed to coincide with the natural surge of luteinizing hormone (LH) that triggers the final maturation of the eggs and ovulation (see page 10). With IVF, the eggs are retrieved (see page 173) 36 hours after the HCG injection, after the final maturation but just before ovulation.

At the end of stimulation, most of the follicles should vary in size from 18–23mm (½–¾in) in diameter, but at this stage it is impossible to tell whether or not there is an egg that can be collected from every follicle. Sometimes the follicle develops at a faster rate than the egg, so when it comes to egg collection the egg is so immature it cannot be removed. And it is quality, of course, not quantity, that counts when it comes to eggs. About 90 per cent of visible follicles of the right size produce a collectable egg, but a substantial number of eggs

does not necessarily mean that they will all be of good quality. On average, about 7–12 eggs are collected from among the 10–20 follicles that started to ripen at the beginning of the cycle.

The short protocol

This protocol is also known as the boost or flare regime. The short protocol takes advantage of the natural flare in FSH and LH levels around day two or three of your cycle, which stimulates follicles to develop. A suppression drug that has the same effect as gonadotrophin-releasing hormone (GnRH) – see page 167 – is given on day two of the cycle to prevent premature ovulation.

In contrast to the long protocol, which waits 10–12 days for you to be down-regulated before starting stimulation drugs, the short protocol prescribes FSH injections the next day (day 3). From here on, the two protocols are the same (see under Monitoring your progress, page 169).

Managing injections

You will be expected to administer the injections yourself – the clinic will give you clear instructions. If you doubt you will be able to manage this, talk to your clinic about organizing a way of having it done under medical supervision. For most women, self-injection becomes easier with practise: a few times is usually enough for them to become confident. You might find the following useful:

* Allow plenty of time for your first few injections. If you are working, prioritize this time and make sure nothing infringes upon it.
* Get your partner involved, as long as he's not too squeamish. Many partners overcome their initial nervousness to become experts at giving injections.
* Sometimes the site of the injection can feel hot. A dab of aloe vera is soothing and cooling
* Apply arnica cream if bruises start to form.
* Warm up the area to be injected first by rubbing the skin or applying a hot-water bottle. This will make it easier to get the needle in.

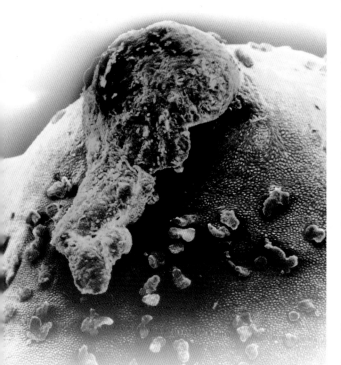

Follicular fluid (blue) is expelled as a mature follicle, lying beneath the swollen surface of the ovary, ruptures at ovulation. The ovum is in the follicle ready to be ejected into the Fallopian tube.

Feeling the effects

Every woman responds differently to the drugs. Mood swings, tearfulness, general emotional fragility and abdominal bloating are all common symptoms. Remember that this stage does not last for long. Most symptoms will disappear when you have finished the injections. If you have serious concerns, contact your fertility consultant.

I see a lot of anxiety in women, especially around the time of their scans, as they discover how their bodies have responded to treatment.

You are at the mercy of your hormones and for a few days will be riding an emotional roller coaster. You may be difficult to live with and your partner may find it impossible to say or do the right thing. Accept the fact that you will have good days and bad. You each need to observe these mood swings objectively and rationally for what they are instead of falling prey to them. Bear in mind that at any point the treatment may not go according to plan. And if the response is poor, it may mean that the cycle has to be abandoned.

Q&A

* What if I have a poor response?

About 10 per cent of women do not respond to stimulation, which means oestrogen levels are low and follicles are not growing. The definition of "poor response" varies from clinic to clinic. It is important to check follicle-stimulating hormone (FSH) levels at the beginning of a cycle before treatment to get an indication of how you will respond. Careful monitoring will allow the drug dosage to be increased or reduced as necessary. If you respond poorly, don't give up hope. A first IVF cycle is very much a case of trial and error, finding out how you will respond and what combinations of drugs suit you best. It isn't always possible to get it right first time. Talk to your doctor about varying the drugs next time or, if necessary, try another clinic.

* What happens if my ovaries are stimulated too much?

Some degree of over-stimulation occurs in all women going through this procedure because the drugs are making the ovaries ripen as many eggs at one time as occurs in more than a year of normal ovulation. If more than 30 follicles are stimulated, you may have ovarian hyperstimulation syndrome (OHSS) – see below.

If your doctor is concerned that too many follicles have grown and your oestradiol level is high, you may be left to "coast". The HCG injection will be withheld, the stimulation drugs stopped and suppression continued. You will be closely monitored. Get plenty of bed rest and drink lots of water at this time.

Occasionally, the ovaries become massively enlarged and fluid starts to build up in the abdomen and thorax. This is ovarian hyperstimulation syndrome (OHSS). Symptoms include:

* severe pain in the lower abdomen and bloating
* breathing difficulties
* nausea and vomiting
* faintness
* reduced urination.

In extreme cases, OHSS can result in thrombosis, heart attack or stroke. The condition can develop quickly, which is why regular monitoring at this stage of the IVF procedure is so important. Familiarize yourself with the symptoms of OHSS and contact a hospital immediately if you experience any of them.

* What happens if the lining of the uterus does not thicken enough?

By the time of egg collection, your uterine lining should be about 9–10mm thick (about a third of an inch) – see page 12. Poor uterine lining may be the result of a previous infection in the uterus (see pages 108–11), fibroids (see pages 117–19) or the repeated use of clomiphene (see page 151). If the endometrium does not thicken adequately during the stimulation programme, it will be very difficult for an embryo to embed. I often use acupuncture at this time to improve blood flow to the endometrium.

Zita's tips

* **Your main aim** is to grow eggs, so concentrate all your efforts and visualization on this. Try to stay relaxed and take each day as it comes. Getting over-anxious about the results of scans and tests will release adrenaline into your bloodstream, which may counter the effects of the drugs you take.

* **Go to bed early.** Never underestimate the power of sleep and rest to enable the body to adapt, repair and grow.

* **Rest is vitally important.** Lie down and put your feet up whenever you can. Exercise and activity directs blood to your extremities, whereas you want it to feed your uterus and the eggs. Even just sitting at a desk or driving a car restricts the flow of energy to the abdomen.

Grapefruit, lemon or lime essential oil in a warm bath will relax you and lift your spirits.

* **Make a conscious decision** to get rid of negative thoughts as they arise. Repeat positive affirmations out loud, even if it makes you feel as though you are a bit eccentric: "My eggs are growing and ripening and maturing; my eggs are of good quality; my womb lining is growing thick".

* **Use visualization** to try and bring about what you are trying to achieve (see page 43). Imagine that you are directing the delivery of oxygen to the lining of your uterus, helping it to develop. Try to visualize the eggs growing. Focus on how you want your body to respond and use these positive images to help you banish fear. This technique also helps you to sit quietly and relax, and it improves the flow of blood and therefore the supply of energy around the body.

* **Avoid stressful situations.** Spend some time each day sitting quietly and breathing slowly and deeply. Use breathing techniques (see pages 42–43) to encourage blood flow through the uterus.

* **Make sure your diet** includes lots of protein (see pages 55–56), which will improve egg quality.

* **Take a daily supplement** of DHA (see pages 63–64) to encourage the development of cell membranes.

* **Take a good general vitamin and mineral supplement,** but one containing vitamin E and co-enzyme Q10 (see pages 61 and 63).

* **Drink plenty of water.** 1–2 litres (1.75–3.5 pints) a day keeps you hydrated. Avoid alcohol, coffee, tea and other stimulants.

* **Try regular acupuncture** with an experienced practitioner (see pages 72–73). There is research to suggest that acupuncture may stimulate the follicles to grow.

* **Keep your lower abdomen warm,** using a hot-water bottle for example. In Chinese medicine, warmth is considered necessary for blood flow.

Egg collection and transfer

The egg retrieval procedure varies from one clinic to another, but you are most likely to be either heavily sedated or given a general anaesthetic. This stage may be a source of anxiety for you.

What is the procedure?

Retrieval of the eggs from the follicles is generally done using a vaginal ultrasound probe, which guides a needle to aspirate each follicle in order to collect eggs. Most clinics will give you a sedative.

The length of time egg retrieval takes depends on the number of follicles, but it is not a lengthy procedure. Once the egg has been aspirated from the follicle, it is carefully inspected under a microscope and given a grading (see page 175). You will be anxious to know how many eggs have been obtained, but it is quality, not quantity, that matters. Not all the eggs will be fertilized, so the number retrieved is no indication of how many embryos there might be in the end.

On the evening after retrieval (or on the day of the transfer, depending on the clinic) you will start taking progesterone, either by vaginal or anal suppository or injection. This prepares the uterine lining to receive the embryo. If your pregnancy is positive, you will take it for up to 12 weeks, again depending on the clinic. Common side effects include nausea, constipation and fluid retention. Antibiotics will also be given to you after the retrieval.

Sperm collection

Your partner will now have to produce sperm ready to fertilize the eggs, having abstained from sexual intercourse for two days. Providing a sperm sample at the clinic can be a stressful experience for a man (see page 133). In extreme circumstances it may be possible to produce a sample at home, but you must be able to get the sample to the clinic immediately for preparation for the next stage of the procedure.

Fertilization

Fertilization protocols also vary from clinic to clinic, but a decision will already have been made about the best fertilization option for you. This will mean one of the following:

* **IVF** (in vitro fertilization) Sperm are prepared, washed and counted and then combined with the eggs in a culture medium in a small shallow dish or test tube in the laboratory and incubated. After 18 hours they are examined. If fertilization has occurred, there will be two pro-nuclei – one from the egg and one from the sperm. Within 48 hours, cell division will have begun and the embryo will be ready for transferral.

Q&A

* **How will I feel after retrieval?**
  You will feel a little groggy from the sedative and your abdomen may be swollen and sore. You might also experience some cramping but this will pass within 24 hours. There is a slight risk of hyperstimulation if a large number of follicles have been emptied and they fill up with fluid (see OHSS in the box on page 171). Contact a doctor immediately if you start to develop symptoms.

* **Is it normal to have spotting after retrieval?**
  You may experience bright red vaginal spotting for 24–48 hours, caused by puncture wounds in the vagina. If bleeding develops, call the clinic immediately.

* **What can go wrong at this stage?**
  The biggest problem at this stage of the procedure will be the failure of the sperm to fertilize the eggs.

Zita's tips

Before retrieval

* **Take the homeopathic remedy** Arnica (6c potency) four times a day starting the day before the procedure, to help prevent soreness and bruising. Continue until after transferral.

* **Take supplements of DHA** (see pages 63–64 and 162) and vitamins C and E (see pages 61 and 162), and eat plenty of foods rich in iron (see page 61).

* **Acupuncture** (see pages 72–73) can help to prepare the endometrium ready to receive the embryos and assist the healing process.

* **Practise breathing techniques** to help you to relax during the retrieval process. As you inhale, imagine the breath going to your solar plexus. As you exhale, imagine all the stress and worry that you are experiencing as well as any physical discomfort you have being expelled from the body.

* **Spend 20 minutes** each morning and evening repeating positive affirmations, telling yourself that everything is going according to plan. Refuse to dwell on "what if..." speculation or possible negative outcomes.

Following retrieval

* **Rest as much as you can** in preparation for the placing of the embryos in the uterus. Rest will aid recovery and healing.

* **Take a co-enzyme Q10 supplement** (see page 63), which will help to improve blood flow after retrieval.

* **Visualize** the healing of the ruptured follicles following egg collection and the thickening of the endometrium ready to receive an embryo.

* **Practise deep breathing** and relaxation techniques (see pages 42–43) to encourage a good flow of blood and energy around the body.

* **ICSI** (intra-cytoplasmic sperm injection) A single sperm is injected into the egg under a microscope using a fine glass needle. This is the technique generally used when:
  * the sperm have poor motility and cannot penetrate the egg; when the sperm count is too low for IVF; when there is a very high proportion of abnormal sperm; or when there are very high levels of antibodies in the semen
  * the sperm has to be surgically obtained
  * there has been a poor rate of fertilization, or none at all, with previous IVF attempts. You can normally expect a fertilization rate of 60–70 per cent. Some eggs will not be successfully fertilized because they are too immature, too ripe or of poor quality generally; some eggs might be fertilized by defective sperm; and not all eggs that are fertilized will go on to divide. Fertilization may, of course, fail to occur at all.
* **IMSI** (intra-cytoplasmic morphologically selected sperm injection) A variation of ICSI that uses a higher-powered microscope to select sperm. Embryologists look at the sperm in greater detail, and then sperm with the most normally shaped nuclei are selected. Studies have shown that selecting better-shaped sperm can improve ICSI outcomes.

Embryo grading

You will, at this stage of the IVF procedure, be very interested in the quality and development of

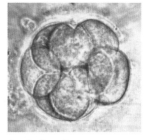

Grade 1 embryo: even cell division, an appropriate number of cells for the culture time and no fragmentation.

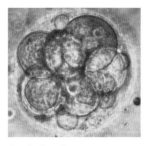

Grade 2 embryo: even cell division and a small amount of fragmentation (extra-cellular debris) between cells.

your embryos and you will probably want regular progress reports. Remember that the grading of the embryos does not correspond directly to your chances of becoming pregnant. High-grade embryos show a tendency to higher pregnancy rates, but they are not a guarantee. I have treated couples whose grading was high-quality but who failed to achieve a successful pregnancy, and I have known couples who were dependent on one frozen embryo and went on to have a baby.

Grading helps to determine how many embryos should be transferred, but it is not an exact science. Try to be positive about your embryos, regardless of their grading, and have faith in the decisions of your medical team. Multi-cell embryos are usually graded from 1–4 (see below), where grade one is best. Sometimes, however, four is best. Your embryos are likely to be of different grades.

Time-lapse monitoring of embryos

EEVA (early embryo viability assessment) uses time-lapse imaging to monitor embryos while they are being incubated, and then uses computer software to select the best embryos at low risk of defects. Pictures taken at five-minute intervals by the computer enable embryologists to check developmental patterns and therefore select the embryos that have a greater viability and most likely to deliver a full pregnancy. In standard IVF, embryos are removed from the incubator once a day to be checked under a microscope.

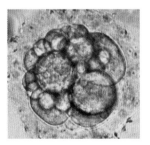

Grade 3 embryo: slightly uneven cell division with a lot of fragmentation between cells.

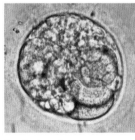

Grade 4 embryo: uneven cell division and excessive amounts of fragmentation between cells.

Pre-implantation genetic screening

A technology called Array CGH is now available to test all 23 chromosomes in a single cell. A major cause of failure of embryos to implant or miscarry is chromosomal abnormality in the embryos. Array CGH makes it possible to screen eggs or embryos so that only chromosomally normal embryos will be selected for transfer into the uterus, thereby improving the chances of successful implantation and reducing the risk of miscarriage. Array CGH may be particularly beneficial for women over 35, and couples experiencing recurrent miscarriage or recurrent IVF failure.

Embryo development

To help you visualize what is happening to your embryos in an attempt to encourage the process to be successful, it might help to know how an embryo develops.

* **Day 1** The first cell division, or cleavage, takes place 33–36 hours after insemination. The eggs are checked to see if fertilization has occurred, identified by the presence of two pro-nuclei. The fused egg and sperm nuclei are known as a zygote, or early embryo.

* **Day 2** At this stage the embryo usually consists of between 2–4 cells. The second cell division takes place 45–46 hours after insemination.

* **Day 3** The third cell division takes place about 54–56 hours after insemination. By this stage, the embryo has 6–8 cells. The individual cells that make up an embryo are known as blastomeres.

* **Day 4** Compaction (when cells start to merge together) occurs and the embryo is known as a morula.

* **Day 5** The embryo now has many cells and develops a fluid-filled cavity. Now it is a blastocyst.

Q&A

* Which drugs accompany this stage?
Most clinics will prescribe progesterone or HCG (human chorionic gonadotrophin) – the hormone that is produced once the placenta attaches – to prepare the uterine lining to accept a fertilized egg and provide support for a developing embryo. Heparin, ritalin or aspirin are also prescribed by some clinics to help blood flow.

* How many embryos should I transfer?
If you are under 40, a maximum of one or two embryos are allowed to be transferred, since the danger of complications rises significantly with a multiple pregnancy. If you are over 40, a maximum of three embryos can be used. Talk to the clinic about this early on so that you feel comfortable with the decision before it is time to transfer.

* What happens to embryos that are not transferred?
Most clinics can freeze embryos and store them for about five years to use in other IVF cycles. The live birth rate per cycle from frozen embryos, however, is usually lower than from fresh embryo transfers.

* Is bed-rest recommended after transfer?
Yes. It will not guarantee a pregnancy, but gives the embryos a better chance of implanting. Activity diverts blood to your extremities and vital organs, whereas lying down allows blood to flow to the endometrium. Do not feel guilty about taking time off work or staying in bed.

* When does implantation occur?
An embryo reaches the blastocyst stage five days after fertilization and starts to break out of its outer shell during the following 48 hours. Only then can it implant. How soon this happens after transfer depends on the stage of the embryo.

* Which factors affect implantation?
The embryos must be of good quality, the endometrium needs to have thickened and your body must not have an immunological reaction to the embryos.

Transferring embryos

This procedure happens between 48 hours and five days after fertilization, depending on what you and your fertility specialist have decided. It is quite an achievement to have got this far, so think positively and try to ignore your inevitable anxiety as you progress to the next stage. Always keep in mind that nothing is certain and it is possible to beat the odds. I have seen successful pregnancies result from low-grade embryos, from frozen embryos and from poor-quality sperm.

Your embryos will be loaded into a small, flexible catheter that will be inserted through the vagina and cervix into the uterus. Ideally you should have an empty bladder, so avoid drinking too much liquid on the morning of the transfer. Some clinics map out your uterus in advance; others use an abdominal ultrasound to guide embryos into place, in which case your bladder needs to be full. When the catheter is in the optimum position near the top of the uterus, the embryos are expelled and the catheter slowly removed. It is then checked back at the lab to make sure that there are no embryos sticking to it.

Keeping calm

The smoother the transfer, the greater the chance of success. Lying on your back for a clinical procedure may well contribute to your anxiety. The adrenaline released by the body in response to the stress you are experiencing may cause the uterus to contract, which will not be helpful to the procedure. So use relaxation techniques such as deep breathing, visualization or meditation (see pages 42–43) to calm yourself down. If you are able to watch what is taking place on a screen, it will give you a better idea of what is happening to your embryos and make visualization easier.

It may be reassuring to have your partner along with you for the transfer, but don't insist upon it if he is reluctant. You need someone to help you reduce stress levels during the procedure, not contribute to them.

The two-week wait

Remember that to have come this far is fantastic considering all of the other hurdles you have had to negotiate. I believe that women have forgotten how to convalesce – you have been through a lot so give yourself time!

The waiting game

There will be good days and bad days over the next two weeks as, full of anxiety, hope and a desperate longing to know if you're pregnant or not, you ride yet another emotional roller coaster. Allow yourself to be optimistic. Even if this is not your first IVF cycle, you are bound to feel a sense of anticipation. Try to banish negative thoughts and repeat to yourself – "I *am* pregnant. This *is* working".

Days 1–4

After all the regular scans and tests, you may feel at a bit of a loose end and cut off. You should ring the clinic at any time if you are concerned. A friend can be a great support, especially if your partner is adopting a pragmatic "either it's worked or it hasn't" attitude. You could use an IVF website or chatroom to "talk" to other women who are going through the same experience.

Rest and relaxation "Carry your embryos with pride", one woman once said to me. Don't feel guilty about taking time off work and lying in bed. You will want to be very careful with yourself. Rest and sleep will give your body the best chance to repair and take the course you want it to. At the very least, lie on the sofa with your feet up as often as possible. Watch DVDs back-to-back; read books. Equally, you shouldn't feel guilty if you do have to return to work.

Your body prepares for the implantation of an embryo with a cycle of hormonal stimulation. The endometrium thickens and the site of implantation becomes swollen with a supply of new blood capillaries. The Chinese believe that if you focus your mind on a particular area in your body, *qi* or life energy will flow to that spot. So, spend 15–20 minutes every morning and evening visualizing what is going on inside your uterus – the embryos are floating safely and are ready to embed in the endometrium, which is thick and well prepared.

In Traditional Chinese Medicine, the kidneys play an important role in reproduction. They may quickly become depleted of energy during an IVF cycle. The kidneys are particularly active from 5–7pm so make sure you rest quietly then. Deep breathing will help you relax and enhance the supply of oxygen reaching your uterus.

Other measures Certain essential oils used in burners or candles can help to lift your mood or soothe and calm you. Try lavender for relaxation; lemon, lime or grapefruit to raise your spirits; or jasmine if you are feeling low. Alternatively, the flower remedy (see page 147) mimulus may help if you are feeling overly anxious about the outcome of your egg transfer. If you are finding it difficult to relax, try white chestnut flower remedy. If you are haunted by past failures, take walnut.

What not to do

During the two-week wait, you must avoid:
* caffeine, tobacco, alcohol, drugs
* heavy lifting
* strenuous exercise, including housework
* bouncing activities, such as horse riding or aerobics
* sun bathing, saunas, hot tubs, jacuzzis, hot baths
* swimming
* sexual intercourse.

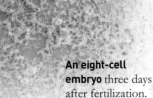

breasts, mild shooting pains and bloating are all indications, in fact, that things are going well.

It's very important to keep yourself occupied. Go for a leisurely walk or do some gentle yoga. Focus on the colour blue if you feel yourself starting to panic. Practise deep breathing and meditation (see pages 42–43) to help you relax. Talk your worries through with a friend or your partner but focus on the positive.

You might like to consider acupuncture (see pages 72–73) seven days following transfer or other relaxing techniques. Try and imagine the embryo embedding in the thickened endometrium. Ideally it will implant on the back wall of the uterus. New blood capillaries then start to develop and the placenta begins to form. The cells in the embryo continue to divide rapidly, forming a two-layered disc, the top layer of which will become the embryo and the amniotic cavity, and the lower of which will be the yolk sac.

Days 8–14

The waiting game seems to be going on for ever. Even if you have gone back to work, you must still try to take things easy and avoid any stressful situations. Only do light tasks and rest as much as you possibly can. Spend your free time seeing friends or plan a long weekend away rather than doing lots of things around the house.

Acupuncture may be beneficial at this stage to boost your kidneys. Make sure you see an acupuncturist who has experience of treating women who are pregnant as a result of IVF treatment. Interestingly, one of the relevant acupoints treated on the kidney meridian is called the Gate of Life (see page 73).

There are a number of other complementary treatments you might like to try at this point. Have a massage, but make sure you visit a qualified practitioner and tell them about the treatment you have been having. Meditate for at least 20 minutes every day. Do lots of positive visualization.

An eight-cell embryo three days after fertilization.

Keep the lower abdomen warm – I cannot stress this enough – but stop using a hot-water bottle once you have had the transfer. Remember that you cannot "grow" a baby if this part of the body is cold. Eat warm, nourishing food.

Finally, make sure your diet is rich in protein, zinc and essential fatty acids (see pages 55–56 and 59–64). Take a good multivitamin and mineral supplement and DHA. Eat foods that are rich in selenium (see page 63), and remember to drink a minimum of 1–2 litres (1.75–3.5 pints) of water a day.

Days 5–7

You may be starting to get restless, obsessively thinking about the implantation, looking for signs that things are going according to plan and possibly misinterpreting every symptom. Sore

By all means take some exercise, but try to keep it low-key, such as leisurely walking, gentle yoga postures, tai chi or qi gong. Avoid all forms of aerobic exercise.

Pregnancy testing

The only way you can be sure whether or not you are pregnant is to have a blood test – an HCG (human chorionic gonadotrophin) or beta blood test – at your fertility clinic. If you decide to use a home testing kit (which I know, in reality, many women will not be able to resist doing), make sure not to use it too early – it might give you an agonizingly misleading result.

HCG is the hormone that starts being produced as soon as the embryo attaches to the endometrium (see page 12). The level doubles every 48 hours in the first weeks of pregnancy, and then continues to in the weeks after that. The level peaks at about 8–10 weeks then declines and remains at a lower level until term.

Even the most sensitive blood test cannot detect HCG until about ten days after ovulation, and there is huge variation in what is regarded as the "normal" level. Pregnancies that eventually miscarry or which are ectopic often show normal HCG levels initially, whereas low levels may still produce a healthy pregnancy.

So, do try not to resort to using a home testing kit too early, and be guided by your fertility clinic.

Getting the results

If the result of your pregnancy test is positive, many congratulations! Your longed-for goal has been realized at last. Take a moment to absorb the information, relax and then celebrate. Be prepared, however, for the development of conflicting emotions as you think about what lies ahead. Many women feel a bit lost because they suddenly have no medication to take or doctors to visit. Nurture yourself (see page 181), especially if you have been anxious.

Case history

Elizabeth, aged 26, was diagnosed with polycystic ovary syndrome (PCOS) after her periods stopped. She took the contraceptive pill until she got married, but then found her periods stopped again. After a year she sought help and was prescribed clomiphene. The next three months she describes as "absolutely horrific. I couldn't sleep, I was tearful; it was like having bad PMS all the time".

It became clear that Elizabeth was still not ovulating. She felt very discouraged and "ready to give up" the idea of having a baby altogether. A friend of hers recommended that she came to me for acupuncture treatment. I referred her on for further fertility testing. Following a hysteroscopy and laparoscopy, which confirmed that Elizabeth was not ovulating, she decided to opt for IVF. "I felt bloated and hormonal when I started the treatment, but I just had to get on with it."

Elizabeth's first cycle of IVF was successful but, sadly, she lost her baby at seven weeks. Four months later she began a second cycle and is now pregnant again. "The whole experience has brought my husband and I much closer together and has made this pregnancy even more special."

Dealing with a negative result

If the result of your pregnancy test is negative, do not despair. Don't try to put on a brave face: accept the fact that you feel devastated. Many of my clients who have received a negative test result report that a failed IVF cycle resembles a mini miscarriage, with exactly the same feelings of loss and grief. Allow yourself time to mourn the collapse of your dream of a baby this month. Take a few days off work if necessary. Be antisocial if you want to be. It will be hard to imagine at the time, but you will feel stronger after a few weeks.

Although you may feel at your lowest ebb right now, the experience you have just been through has by no means been a waste of time. Your clinic will have learned a great deal about you and your physiology that will enable them to make adjustments to the treatment programme if there is going to be a next time. If you are keen to have another try, arrange a meeting with your fertility consultant and talk about what has been learned and what could be done differently next time.

I have seen very many women go on to conceive at their next attempt at IVF, after they have taken three months off for rest and recuperation, physical as well as mental. If, however, you feel you have reached the end of the road and you cannot put yourself through it again, talk to your doctor about other options, but always try to keep an open mind. You might change it.

Zita's tips

* **The second week is the worst** One minute you will be fairly sure that the treatment has worked and you have conceived a baby, but the next minute you will be plunged into despair, convinced that it hasn't worked and your period is imminent.

* **You will feel very hormonal** Emotional fragility may make you feel very vulnerable and as if you have no control over your fate.

* **Reading the signs** Remember that every woman's experience is different. There is no standard set of symptoms that you get as side effects of all the drugs you have been taking, or as you recover from the IVF cycle or during the early stages of pregnancy (see opposite) for that matter. Whatever the "signs" are, you will probably be just as able to translate them negatively as positively, depending on the mood you are in at the time. You may have no symptoms at all, but you might have bloating and fluid retention, breast tenderness, drowsiness and exhaustion, slight cramping, PMS symptoms, night sweats, aversions to certain foods, nausea and slight bleeding or a brownish discharge. If you are not pregnant, you may start to bleed before two weeks after transfer.

* **Stay focused on your goal** Continue to practise relaxation techniques, meditate and visualize positive outcomes. Don't look too far ahead, stay in the present and take each day as it comes. Banish negative thoughts as they arise and only listen to stories and read statistics if you can deal with them, whatever they are, without over-reacting.

* **Seeing babies** You may find there is a recurrence of the phenomenon you experienced as you set out down the road to conception — seeing pregnant women or people with babies everywhere you look!

* **After a negative result** Don't make any rash decisions. If you want to have another go at IVF, your initial instinct may be to make a fresh start at another clinic. Listen to what your consultant has to say about the recent attempt, however, before you make up your mind, and don't forget how many factors you had to weigh up carefully before you made a choice in the beginning. Take time out before you decide.

Pregnancy following IVF

Receiving the longed-for "positive" result of a pregnancy test may have seemed like an end in itself. Finding out that you are expecting a baby, however, may just be the start of a whole new wave of anxieties – about how best to prevent a miscarriage and maintain the pregnancy – as well as a source of deep joy.

Thinking pregnant

It can be really difficult to let go of what has gone before and think of yourself with confidence as a pregnant woman. Take each day at a time and remember that the odds of your pregnancy being successful improve with every week that goes by. Anxiety tends to be a much more common feature of pregnancy following IVF. Every twinge or ache or pain can be a source of worry.

Getting to the 12th week is the first big hurdle. The fetal heartbeat has usually been detected by this point. Your doctor will listen for it using an ultrasound device as part of a routine antenatal check. 94 per cent of pregnancies carry through to a positive conclusion once the fetal heartbeat has been picked up.

A trans-vaginal scan will ensure that your pregnancy is not ectopic. There is a higher risk of an ectopic pregnancy following IVF because the embryos float around for longer before implanting. Try to limit the number of trans-vaginal scans you have and opt for abdominal scans instead.

Taking care

Many women who have been through IVF feel terribly sick in early pregnancy. Welcome this as a good sign and expect to feel exhausted – in other words, feel good about feeling bad. But if you don't feel bad, don't worry! Bear in mind the following:

* Spotting or a slight brownish discharge is normal and nothing to worry about. If bleeding gets heavier, call your clinic immediately.

* Avoid caffeine, alcohol, tobacco, strenuous exercise and hot baths, just as you did during the post-transfer period (see also page 177), and drink 1–2 litres (1.75–3.5 pints) of water a day.

* I advise couples not to have sex for the first 12 weeks of pregnancy if they can possibly avoid it.

* Get plenty of rest and early nights. Take time off work if you need to. Right now, maintaining your pregnancy is more important than anything else.

* Consider a course of acupuncture to replenish and build up energy in the kidneys. Acupuncture has also been shown to be effective in helping to relieve nausea and sickness.

* Don't fly.

Zita's tips

To relieve nausea and sickness in early pregnancy:

* **Eat small, frequent meals**, avoiding spicy or fatty foods. Take a good multivitamin and mineral supplement to ensure that you are not deficient in vitamin B6, magnesium or zinc.

* **Be sure to get as much rest** as you can during the day and as much sleep as possible at night since fatigue and severe sickness seem to be linked.

* **Stimulate the Pericardium 6 acupoint** on your forearm, three finger-widths above the wrist crease between the two tendons. Apply gentle pressure for ten minutes four times a day.

Looking at other options

If diagnosis and treatment have ruled out the possibility
of having your own child, you need to ask yourselves some
important questions. Can you accept that only one partner
is a biological parent? Should you consider adoption?

Sperm donation

If your partner is producing no sperm at all, or if
he is at risk of passing on a genetic disorder, donor
insemination (DI) may be the only way that you
as a couple can have a child. The use of sperm
from anonymous donors is licensed by the Human
Fertilization and Embryology Authority (HFEA).
DI is being used less with the success of micro-
manipulation techniques such as ICSI and IMSI
(see page 174), which enable men who have very
low sperm counts to fertilize their partners' eggs.

Donors are rigorously screened and can be
matched to your partner for race, build, colouring
and blood group. Greater openness about donors
should help to reassure you both. "Quarantining"
procedures also ensure your safety. Donated sperm
is thoroughly tested for HIV and a variety of
infections before being frozen and quarantined for
six months. It is thawed immediately before use.

Your cycle will be monitored by temperature
monitoring, an ovulation prediction kit or ultrasound
scans and, if necessary, you will be given fertility
drugs to ensure ovulation. Insemination occurs at
ovulation, when sperm are placed in the vagina,
cervix or uterus. If several cycles do not produce
a result, DI may be combined with IVF.

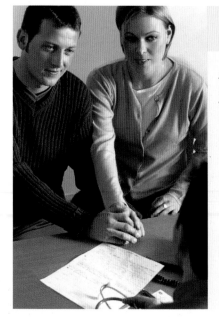

What you need to know about DI

Although donor insemination may be the next logical step, it has
psychological and emotional implications, particularly for your partner, who
will be having a child that is not genetically his. Consider the following
before you make a final decision.

* **You must both take the time to talk** about all the issues involved. Don't
  pressurize your partner if he isn't keen – DI must be right for both of you.

* **Counselling is essential** because of potential ethical, legal and social
  problems. Both you and your partner's written consent is needed,
  including your partner's consent to become the legal father of any
  child born as a result of treatment.

* **Anonymous donors must remain so by law** and they have no rights
  over children conceived and born using their sperm.

* **Your decision to opt for donor insemination remains private.** You
  don't have to tell anybody and nobody else need ever know.

Egg donation

Egg donation is an increasingly common option and may be one you should consider. If you are not producing eggs, perhaps because of an inherited condition, surgery, chemotherapy, ovarian disease or early menopause, the only way you may be able to conceive and carry a child yourself is by using donated eggs. This is also an option for women over 40 whose egg quality is declining and for women who are at risk of passing on a genetic disorder to their offspring. If you use a donated egg, you and your partner will still be able to bond with the baby throughout your pregnancy and the birth. Half your baby's genes will belong to your partner and you will both be the baby's legal parents. As with sperm donation, however, you do as a couple need to think long and hard about all the issues involved.

Both you and the donor must, by law, be given counselling to help you consider fully all the emotional, social, medical, legal and ethical issues surrounding egg donation. You need to consider, for example, how and when you will tell your child about his or her genetic origins. As with donor insemination, your decision to use donor eggs can remain private and nobody else need ever know.

What is involved?

The donor has to go through the IVF cycle as far as egg collection. The donated eggs are then fertilized by your partner's sperm and the resulting embryo frozen until you are ready for it to be transferred. It may be at once if your cycle has been manipulated to match that of the donor.

IVF success rates with egg donation cycles tend to be higher than with routine IVF, because the eggs are all from women under the age of 35, and you (the recipient) have not gone through super-ovulation drug treatment. This means that your endometrium is in a more natural state of receptivity, although you may be given oestrogen to encourage implantation. On the other hand, egg donation can be emotionally stressful and you will have to deal with the uncertainty about whether or not the donor will produce enough eggs.

Many women seeking egg donation go overseas, as the donors are anonymous. If you have egg donation in the UK, the donor can be traced. Egg donors cannot be paid in the UK other than for their travel expenses. Waiting lists are long. Although a relative can be a donor, you are more likely to be using an anonymous donor who will be matched as closely as possible with you for race, type and characteristics. She will be screened for viral conditions and genetic disorders.

You need to think long and hard about the complex issues involved in egg donation and be sure you are both completely happy with your decision.

Moving on

"How will I know when it's time to give up and move on?" That's the million-dollar question I get asked time and time again. The answer is, of course, different for every couple.

Coming to a conclusion

The decision that you are ready to give up the chance to have your own biological child is possibly the one stage in the process of planning for a baby that is the least predictable. If you have fertility problems and have been undergoing treatment, you will keep moving the goalposts until you reach the point at which you realize that enough is enough and you have gone as far as you are prepared to go. It is possible for almost every couple to have a baby if they really want one. It is a question of how far they are prepared to move the goalposts as they deal with their fertility problems and, perhaps at the end of a long treatment road, they consider options such as egg donation, surrogacy or the adoption of a child.

You won't know exactly when this realization is going to dawn until it occurs. The factors conspiring to bring about the decision might include:

* your age next birthday
* whether or not you think your relationship can withstand any more of the pressures of trying to have a baby of your own
* whether or not you have the financial resources to pursue any more options
* whether or not you have the emotional strength to keep going
* whether or not you feel as if your body has been through enough
* the advice of your doctors and the predicted odds for success of any further treatment or option.

There is usually a doctor somewhere who, with the best possible intentions, will offer "just one more thing you could try", and it is tempting to hang on to yet another last thread of hope. Don't, however, become so fixed on an endless pursuit that you lose all sense of perspective. Take care not to become so bound up with the quest to become a parent that a sense of failure overshadows all the positive aspects of life, destroying your self-esteem.

Some women wake up one day knowing they have reached the end of the road, and are ready to reclaim their life and their body. They want to stop defining themselves in terms of their fertility and regain a sense of normality. Others realize this gradually. If you and your partner do not get to this point at the same time, you will need to give each other time and support, and you may need counselling to help you do this.

No regrets

It is important, as far as possible, to move on from fertility treatment knowing that "you've given it your best shot", and to be able to look back in five years' time and view the whole experience without any regrets. That means knowing that you:

* made all the necessary nutritional and lifestyle changes that were recommended to you to enhance your fertility
* received the best medical attention that you could afford at the time
* followed the recommendations of your doctors and specialists
* pursued all the treatment options that were appropriate for you and that had a reasonable chance of success
* gave each option your best effort, thinking positively about it and believing in it.

Mixed emotions

You may have made a monumental decision, but the emotional roller coaster of the last few months or years may not be over just yet. Expect to feel some, if not all, of the following:

* **relief** that there are no more tests, scans, injections or other procedures that you will have to endure
* **liberation** from what felt like a never-ending cycle of hope and despair
* **anger** because "this wasn't the way it was all supposed to end"
* **betrayal** because the medical profession has failed, despite all the resources and latest technology at its disposal, to give you the right answers or solutions
* **grief** and a huge sense of loss as you mourn the child you will never have
* **exhaustion**, both physical and emotional
* **strength**, because you've not only survived intact but have grown in the process
* **the freedom** to take back your life and return to some kind of normality
* **hope** as you plan for a new future.

Give yourself as much time as you need to work through each of these emotions. Complete emotional healing and recovery may take years, but it is important to come to terms with some of these feelings as soon as possible. Talking them through with a friend or counsellor and reviewing the road you've travelled along since you first started to think about having a baby can be a very constructive part of the healing process.

What of the future?

You will then be ready to move on and investigate the options of surrogate parenting, adopting, fostering or, of course, child-free living. It is now time to think very carefully about:

* how important is the experience of raising a child to you and your partner?
* how important is the necessity for one of you to have a biological/genetic link to that child?

Make sure that you and your partner understand each other's needs so that the solution you choose suits both of you equally. The more clearly you can identify and fully appreciate your reasons for wanting to be a parent in the first place, the more clearly you will be able to identify the right path forward in the future. As many couples will tell you, there are more ways to create a happy family than by giving birth to a baby.

Case history

Having suffered seven miscarriages over five years and tried four IVF cycles, all of them unsuccessful, Sarah started to think about surrogacy. "The UK provided no answers for me, and I had to conclude that surrogacy is still rather frowned upon here. I began to focus my attention on the United States, where it is a much more acceptable option for women who cannot have a baby of their own." *Sarah decided to pursue a surrogacy programme through an American agency.* "It has proved to be yet another emotional roller coaster. I had slight misgivings about the first surrogate, so I decided not to go ahead. **I was concerned not to act out of desperation but to keep looking until I found someone with whom I felt totally comfortable.** The second attempt has gone well so far. It's still early days but I'm optimistic it will work out."

Further information

REFERENCES

Page 16
Khatamee and Rosenthal, The Fertility Sourcebook, McGraw-Hill Contemporary, 2002

Page 20
Journal of Family Planning and Reproductive Health Care, 2001, 27 (2), 103–10

Page 30
Longscope C G, Orbach S, Goldin B et al, 1987, *Effect of low-fat diet on oestrogen metabolism,* J Clin Endocrinol Metab, 64 (6), 1246–49

Page 31
Arnold S E, Klotz D M, Collins B M et al, 1996, *Synergistic activation of oestrogen receptor with combination of environmental chemicals,* Science, 272, 1489–92;
Baird D, *Smokers face higher infertility,* J Am Med Assoc, 1985, 253, 2979–83;
Bopp B and Shoupe D, 1993, *Luteal Phase Defects,* J Repro Med, May, 38 (5), 348–56; Tuormaa T E, *Adverse effects of alcohol on reproduction: literary review,* International Journal of Biosocial and Medical Research, 14 (2), In press, 1994

Page 33
Wilcox A et al, *Caffeinated beverages and decreased fertility,* The Lancet, Vol 2 (1998), 1453–55

Page 34
Baird D, *Smokers face higher infertility,* J Am Med Assoc, 1985, 253, 2979–83;
Tuormaa T E, *Adverse effects of alcohol on reproduction: literary review,* International Journal of Biosocial and Medical Research, 14 (2), In press, 1994; Ward N et al, *The placental element levels in relation to fetal development of obstetrically normal births. A study of 37 elements. Evidence of the effects of cadmium, lead and zinc on fetal growth, and smoking as a cause of cadmium,* International Journal of Biosocial

Research, Vol 9 (1), 1987, 6308;
Wyn M and Wyn A, *The case for pre-conception for men and women,* AB Academic Publishers (1991)

Page 36
Batzinger R P, Ou S Y L, and Bueding E, *Saccharin and other sweeteners: mutagenic properties,* Science, 1977, 198, 944–46; Fertility and Sterility, vol 71, no 3, March 1999;
Goyer R A, *Lead toxicity: a problem in the environment,* Am J Pathol, 1971, 64, 167–79;
Ondrizek R R, Chan P J, Patton W C, and King A, Department of Gynecology and Obstetrics, Loma Linda University School of Medicine, California, USA, *Inhibition of human sperm motility by specific herbs used in alternative medicine,* J Assist Reprod Genet, 16, 87–91, Feb 1999;
Reif-Lehrer L, *Possible significance of adverse reactions to glutamate in humans,* Federation Proceedings, 1976, 35, 2205–11, 1976
Schroeder H A and Tipton I H, *The human body burden of lead,* Arch Environ Health, 1968, 18, 965–78;

Page 41
Fertility and Sterility, 2001, 76:3, 10–16. ©2001 by American Society for Reproductive Medicine.

Page 46
Grant Ellen, *Sexual Chemistry,* Cedar Press, 1994

Page 47
Farrow A, Hull MGR et al, *Prolonged use of oral contraception before a planned pregnancy is associated with a decreased risk of delayed conception,* Human Reproduction (ALSPAC study), Vol 17, 2002, 10, 2754–61
Gnoth C, Frank-Herrmann P,

Schmoll A et al, *Cycle characteristics after discontinuation of oral contraceptives,* Gynecol Endocrinol, 2002, Aug 16 (4): 307–17
Vessey M P, Smith M A, Yeates D, Oxford, FPA study, *Return of fertility after discontinuation of oral contraceptives – influence of age and parity,* British Journal of Family Planning, 1986, Vol II, 120–40

Page 59
Crawford M A, *The role of dietary fatty acids in biology: their place in the evolution of the human brain,* Nutritional Reviews (1992), 50, 3–11;
Czeizel A E et al, Dept of Human Genetics and Teratology, WHO Collaborating Centre for the Community Control of Hereditary Disease, Budapest, Hungary, *The effect of pre-conceptional multivitamin supplementation on fertility,* International Journal for Vitamin and Nutrition Research, 1996, 66 (1) 55–58;
Shrimpton Derek, *A scientific evaluation of the range of intakes,* commissioned by the European Federation of Health Product Manufacturers' Association and published by the Council for Responsible Nutrition, October 1997;
Olsen F F, *Does fish consumption during pregnancy increase fetal size? A study of the size of newborn, placental weight, gestational age & fish intake,* International Journal of Epidemiology (1990), 19, 971–77

Pages 68 75
Journal of Family Planning and Reproductive Health Care, 2001, 27 (2), 103–10

Page 69
Rex K M et al, *Nocturnal light effects on menstrual cycle length,* Journal of

Complementary Medicine, 1997, 3, 387–90;

Roennburg T and Aschoff J, *Annual rhythm of human reproduction: 11 environmental correlations*, Journal of Biological Rhythms, 1990, 5, 217–39

Pages 72–73

Chen B Y, *Acupuncture normalises dyfunction of hypothalamic-pituitary-ovarian axis*, Acupunct Electrother Res, 1997, 22, 97–108;

Steer C V, Campbell S, Tan S L, Crayford T, Mills C, Mason B A et al, *The use of transvaginal colour flow imaging after in vitro fertilization to identify optimum uterine conditions before embryo transfer*, Fertil Steril, 1992, 57, 372–76;

Stener-Victorin E, Waldenström U, Andersson S A, and Wikland M, *Reduction of blood flow impedance in the uterine arteries of infertile women with electro-acupuncture*, Hum Reprod, 1996, 11 (6), 1314–17;

Stener-Victorin E, Waldenström U, Nilsson L, Wikland M, and Janson P O, *A prospective randomized study of electro-acupuncture versus alfentanil as anaesthesia during oocyte aspiration in in-vitro fertilization*, Hum Reprod, 1999, 14 (10), 2480–84;

Stener-Victorin E, Waldenström U, Tagnfors U, Lundeberg T, Lindstedt G, and Janson P O, *Effects of electro-acupuncture on anovulation in women with polycystic ovary syndrome*, Acta Obstet Gynecol Scand, 2000, 79 (3), 180–88

Page 74

Costa M, Canale D, Filicori M et al, *L-carnitine in idiopathic asthenozoospermia: a multicenter study*, Andrologia, 1994, 26, 155–59;

Dawson E B, Harris W A, Teter M C, and Powell L C, *Effect of ascorbic acid supplementation on the sperm quality of smokers*, Fertil Steril, 1992, 58, 1034–39;

de Aloysio D, Mantuano R, Mauloni M, and Nicoletti G, *The clinical use of arginine aspartate in male infertility*, Acta Eur Fertil, 1982, 13, 133–67;

Fraga C G, Motchnik P A, Shigenaga M K et al, *Ascorbic acid protects against endogenous oxidative DNA damage in human sperm*, Proc Natl Acad Sci, 1991, 88, 11003–06;

Schacter A et al, *Treatment of oligospermia with the amino acid arginine*, Int J Gynaecol Obstet, 1973, 11, 206–09;

Tanimura J, *Studies on arginine in human semen. Part III. The influences of several drugs on male infertility*, Bull Osaka Med School, 1967, 13, 90–100.

Page 109

Morton R F, *Candidal vaginitis natural history predisposing factors and prevention*, Proceedings from the Royal Society of Medicine, Vol 70 (4), 1997, 3–6;

Sutton G, *Genital infections*, Midwife and Health Visitor and Community Nurse, 18 (2), 1982, 42–45;

Weidner W, *Ureaplasmal infections of the male urogenital tract in particular prostatitis and semen quality*, Urology International, Vol 40, 1982, 42–45

Page 113

RS *Microbiology of the female genital tract*, Am Obstet and Gynae, 1987, 156, 491–95

Page 120

Yu J, Zheng M, and Ping S M, *Changes in serum FSH, LH and ovarian follicular growth during electro-acupuncture for induction of ovulation*, Chung Hsi I Cheih Ho Tsa Chih, 1989, 9, 199–202

Page 131

Sliutz G, Speiser P, Schultz A M et al, *Agnus Castus extracts inhibit prolactin secretion of rat pituitary cells*, Horm Metab Re, 1993, 25, 253–55

Page 149

Gravitz M A, *Hypnosis in the treatment of functional infertility*, Am J Clin Hypno, 1995, 38, 22–26;

Hernandez-Reif M, Martinez A, Field T, Quintero O, Hart S, and Burman I, Touch Research Institute, University of Miami School of Medicine, Florida, USA, *Premenstrual symptoms are relieved by massage therapy*, J Psychosom Obstet Gynaecol, Mar 2000, 21 (1), 9–15.

USEFUL WEBSITES

Zita West Clinic
37 Manchester Street, London
W1U 7LJ
Tel: 020 7224 0017
www.zitawest.com

Food Standards Agency
www.food.gov.uk

The Human Fertilization and Embryology Authority (HFEA)
www.hfea.gov.uk

Royal College of Obstetricians and Gynaecologists
www.rcog.org.uk

The British Complementary Medicine Association
www.bcma.co.uk

British Acupuncture Council
www.acupuncture.org.uk

The Miscarriage Association
www.miscarriageassociation.org.uk

TAMBA (Twins & Multiple Births Association)
www.tamba.org.uk

Infertility Network UK
www.infertilitynetworkuk.com

Childlessness Overcome Through Surrogacy UK (COTS)
www.surrogacy.org.uk

Endometriosis UK
www.endometriosis-uk.org

British Nutrition Foundation
www.nutrition.org.uk

IVF websites
www.fertilityfriends.co.uk
www.ivf-infertility.co.uk
www.ivf.net

Index

Acknowledgments

Zita West would especially like to thank Sharon Baylis for helping her to collate the raw material for this book and to write it.
She would also like to thank:
Jude Garlick for her help and enthusiasm over the last six months;
her family – husband Rob, Sofie and Jack;
Vicki McIvor;
Anna Davidson, Anne Esden, Salima Hirani, and Corinne Roberts at DK;
Dr Sheryl Homer for her input on male fertility and IVF;
Jane Knight, Clare Casson, Sally-Anne Caplin, Chew yeen Lawes, Clare Mellon, Joanne Miller and Karen Taylor at her clinic;
Paul Armstrong (Consultant in Obstetrics and Gynaecology), Julia Leonard, Pandora, Bernadette Kelly Rivers, Ian Spiers, Titiana Wait, and Martin Watt.

Dorling Kindersley would like to thank Alyson Lacewing for proof-reading, Sue Bosanko for the index, and picture librarians Hayley Smith and Romaine Werblow. They also thank the following for their kind permission to reproduce their photographs:

1: Getty Images/Paul Vozdic (c); **3**: Getty Images/Sarah Jones (Debut Art); **4-5**: Science Photo Library/ Dr Yorgos Nikas; **6-7**: Getty Images/ Deborah Jaffe; **7**: Jack West; **8-9**: Getty Images/Roz Woodward; **10**: Science Photo Library/Alfred Pasieka (bl), Professor P. M. Motta Et Al (br); **11**: Science Photo Library (bl), Dr Yorgos Nikas (br); **12**: Science Photo Library/Pascal Goetgheluck (b); **13**: Science Photo Library/D. Phillips (cll), Dr Yorgos Nikas (cl), (crr), Professor P. M. Motta & J. Van Blerkom (cr); **15**: Science Photo Library (br); **18**: Corbis/Rick Gomez; **21**: Getty Images/Joe Polillio; **23**: Getty Images/Color Day Production; **25**: Getty Images/Paul Viant; **34**: Getty Images/ Romilly Lockyer; **36**: Getty Images/Eric Larrayadieu; **39**: Getty Images/David Seed Photography; **44**: Getty Images/ V.C.L.; **46**: Getty Images/HOM; **48**: Getty Images/Stephanie Rausser; **50**: Science Photo Library; **54**: Getty Images/Chris Cole; **60**: Getty Images/ Jed & Kaoru Share; **62**: Getty Images /Dennis O'Clair; **65**: Sian Irvine; **69**: Getty Images/David Sacks; **74**: Getty Images/Lori Adamski Peek; **77**: Science Photo Library/Innerspace Imaging; **80**: Getty Images/Ghislain & Marie David de Lossy; **82**: Getty Images/ Anthony Marsland; **83**: Getty Images /Ghislain & Marie David de Lossy; **84**: Getty Images/Alexander Walter (tl), Yorgos Nikas (bc); **85**: Getty Images/Ron Chapple; **86**: Getty Images/Sarah Jones (Debut Art) (br), Werner Bokelberg (tl); **89**: The Wellcome Institute Library, London; **90**: Getty Images/Jerome Tisne (tl); **91**: Corbis/Donna Day (b); **92**: Corbis/Roy Mchon; **94**: Getty Images /Antonio Mo; **97**: Getty Images/Rob Van Petten; **99**: Mother & Baby Picture Library/emap esprit; **100**: Science Photo Library/Professors P. M. Motta & S. Makabe; **103**: Science Photo Library/Nancy Kedersha; **110**: Science Photo Library; **111**: Getty Images/ Romilly Lockyer; **115**: Science Photo Library/Chris Priest; **123**: Getty Images/Zigy Kaluzny; **127**: Getty Images/Ghislain & Marie David de Lossy; **129**: Getty Images/Frederic Tousche; **138**: Getty Images/Color Day Production; **140**: Getty Images/ Romilly Lockyer; **142**: Getty Images /Derek Berwin; **146**: Getty Images/ Michelangelo Gratton (t); **147**: Getty Images/Jim Franco; **148**: Science Photo Library/Cordelia Molloy; **151**: Science Photo Library/Edelman (br); **154**: Getty Images/Oliver Strewe (bl); **157**: Getty Images/Paul Vozdic; **160**: Getty Images/Peter LaMastro; **165**: Getty Images/Gary Buss; **170**: Science Photo Library/Prof. P. Motta /Dept. of Anatomy; **172**: Getty Images/Daniel Bosler; **174**: The Wellcome Institute Library, London /K. Hardy (bc), (br); **175**: The Wellcome Institute Library, London /K. Hardy (bl), (br); **178**: Science Photo Library/Dr Yorgos Nikas; **182**: Mother & Baby Picture Library /emap esprit (bl); **183**: Getty Images /David Harry Stewart.
(Abbreviations key: t=top, b=bottom, r=right, l=left, c=centre)